LOCKDOWN HEALTH

Dr. Prashant. P. Shetty

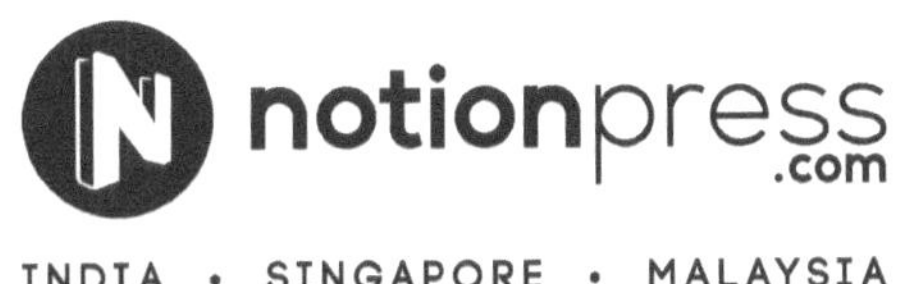

Notion Press

No.8, 3rd Cross Street,
CIT Colony, Mylapore,
Chennai, Tamil Nadu – 600004

First Published by Notion Press 2021
Copyright © Dr. Prashant. P. Shetty 2021
All Rights Reserved.

ISBN 978-1-63806-647-7

Contents

Foreword

The health care sector is undergoing rapid changes all over the world. The problems of the growing elderly population, obesity are on the rise by the day. Though people are realizing it slowly and gradually that to be healthy and fit one doesn't need expensive health care but a deeper understanding of how to eat, exercise, meditation, walking, jogging, running, right food habits and the right attitude towards life. It is here that yoga will be boon for most problems in the 21st century. Yoga became more popular all over the world when India's Prime minister Shri Narendra Modi declared "International yoga day on 21st June.

The Prime Minister in his speech said that "Yoga embodies unity of mind and body; thought and action; restraint and fulfillment; harmony between man and nature; a holistic approach to health and wellbeing."

The present book "LOCKDOWN HEALTH" is an endeavor undertaken by Dr.Prashant.P.Shetty, M.D.S, Ph.D, Professor in Conservative and Endodontics, Pacific Dental College, Debari, Airport road, Udaipur, I wish him all the success.

Dr. Ravikumar CM

Principal

Pacific Dental College & Research Centre,

Bhillo-ka-bedla, Udaipur-313024

Acknowledgement

Reading is passion, writing is action and this book is the outcome of both. Health is a state of complete physical, mental, and social well-being and not merely the absence of disease (WHO). Yoga is ancient science and answer to various modern problems. Yoga is alternative therapies due to its efficacy and cost-effectiveness. Stress is a major cause of a series of diseases leading to a loss in terms of health, money, work hours, and different lifestyles, and Yoga (meditation) is the only solution for this.

I will always remain indebted to our teachers who laid the foundation and were instrumental in shaping my thoughts.

Inspired by the management of the Pacific Group of Institutions, Udaipur, Mr. B.R.Agrawal, Mr. Rahul Agarwal, and Mr. Ashish Agrawal for allowing me to write the book.

It is my great pleasure to express my heartfelt thanks to Dr. A.Bhagwan Das Rai, Principal, Pacific Dental College and Hospital, Debari, Udaipur who always supported and helped me with my endeavour.

Special thanks to Dr. Ravikumar. CM (Principal, Pacific dental College and research center, Bhillo – Ka – Bedla, Udaipur) who was instrumental and ever ready to help when needed.

Thanks to Dr. Bhaskar Rao, Dr. Srinath Thakur (Principal, Sdm dental college, Dharwad) & who guided me when I needed most.

I am equally thankful to Notion Press Publisher for their keen interest and attention in bringing out this book. Special thanks are to

Dr. Madhusudhan Astekar (Hod & Professor, MDS, PhD, Institute of Dental Sciences, Bareilly, Uttar Pradesh. – 243006) for his supporting, enthusiastic assistance and ever ready help during the writing of this book.

I would like to take this opportunity to thank Hod Dr. Sandeep Metgud, Dr. Moulshree Dube, Dr. Deepali Agrawal, Dr. Afzal Ali, Dr. Aseem Jain, postgraduates, undergraduates, alumni and all my dear friends for their help with constant encouragement, love, tolerance and not disturbing me when demanded.

Inspired by my uncle Mr. Vasant Shetty & family who taught me values, to be patient, caring, and supported me in my endeavour. (Kudhi Vasantha Shetty, Headmaster of Vishnumurthy High School at Kudhi village in Udupi district, national-level Best Teacher Award on Teachers Day, at a function held at Rastrapathi Bhavan on Wednesday, September 5, 2012).

I would like to thank Mr. Bhaskar Shetty and family, Dharwad, Late Vijay shetty and Mrs. Suryakanthi Shetty and family, Ninjoor, Udupi, and Mr. Hariprasanna Shetty (MD, Intexso Biochem Pvt. Ltd, Village Hamrapur, Maharashtra-421303) and family for supporting me.

I would like to thank Dr. Dharam Hinduja (HOD, SJM Dental College, Chitradurga, Karnataka) who has always been a great source of inspiration for me.

I would like to thank Manju Kamble (animator of youtube videos fame) Artist, Dharwad for adding colors (Buddha artwork) to this work. I am equally thankful to Mr. Sonu Sharma (Lucky Xerox, Udaipur) for this contribution and timely help in corrections of the book.

Our love, gratitude, and respect to our parents Smt Suma.P.Shetty and Late K.Purandhar Shetty who have always been our pillars of strength throughout our life.

My wife Dr. Preethika Rai, BAMS, M.D in Swasthavrittha,(D.N.Y.S) who wrote about the benefits of different Yoga asanas, Meditation, and weight loss tips, otherwise this would have been impossible. Father in Law Late Madhav Rai, Mother in Law Bhavani Shedthi, my sister Lavanya Shetty (IT ENGINEER and presently working with Tata Consultancy Services, Bangalore) and her son Chinmaya, brother Shashikant shetty (Hotel business, Hubli) and Shyamala bhabhi for their unconditional love, support, wishes and prayers throughout the writing of this book and my life in general for bringing joy into all our lives.

Tons of love to my child Krish who have adjusted according to our work and made it possible to publish the book. Without them, there would be no world to me. I do not have words to thank **The Almighty**, who has protected me and favored me in all aspects through the journey of my life and perhaps much more to pen down my thoughts in the form of a book. Any errors in the book have to be forgiven by the readers. Writing a book requires a significant amount of effort, patience, and sacrifice and at the end of the day, it is worth all the effort if it serves its intended purpose.

I sincerely hope that you enjoy reading **Lockdown Health** and assimilating this book as I have enjoyed writing it. Your opinion, criticism, comments are valuable.

Place: Udaipur   **Dr. Prashant. P. Shetty M.D.S, P.hD**

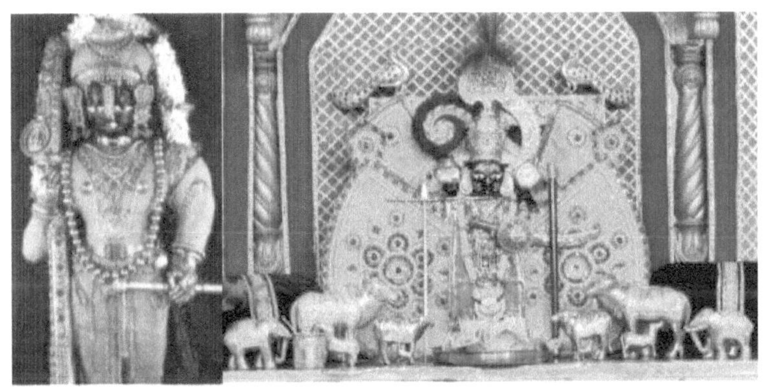

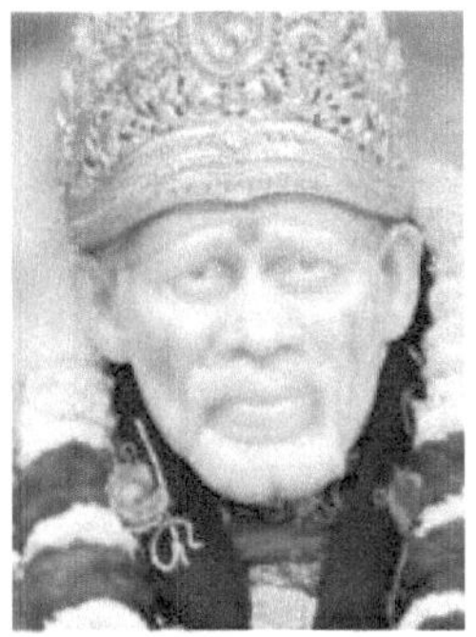

"I am ever living to help and guide all who come to me, who surrender to me"

...Shri Sai Baba

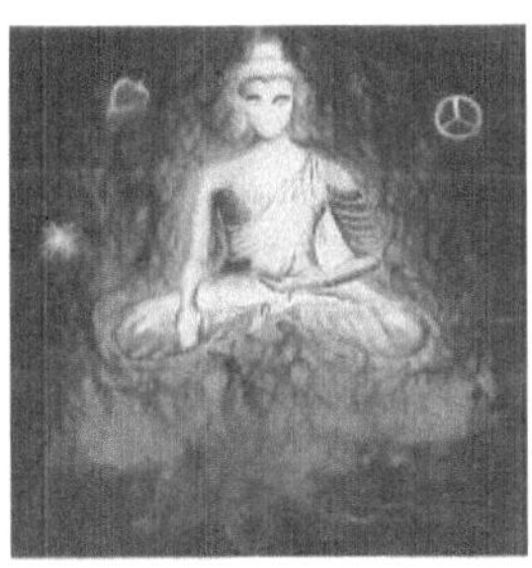

"Don't rush anything. When the time is right, It'll happen."

...Buddha

What This Book Can Do for You?

Of course, we can go on and on with so many ways to reduce weight, what is obesity, exercise to reduce abdomen fat, yoga and out of the box thinking that this book can be titled "Lockdown Health."

But I know that you don't want only that. You want to know how you can get started thinking in your life, to solve your problems and achieve your goals.

You want to know how you can develop your cognitive abilities, so you could generate

more creative ideas and gain an edge over others in terms of providing solutions with regarding health.

This book will change how you perceive your creativity, generate ideas that deliver results, it has the potential to shift the trajectory of your life.

You will perhaps start seeing endless possibilities in front of you. You will learn how to:

Generate ideas on demand for health.

Find new ways to make money by coaching.

Manipulate and modify existing ideas to make them powerful. Create new products, services, and processes.

Develop solutions to complex health problems. See health problems as opportunities.

Become more productive.

Be the "idea person" in your organization.

Know where to look for the "breakthrough idea." and above is just to list a few benefits.

I want to equip you with the most effective strategies that will help you think out of the

box and help you get creative ideas. I know it's a big promise for your body but here is the silver lining. The strategies I will be telling in the book are not something invented by me, rather they are used by the many creative thinkers of the world. Since they have worked out for them, it should work for you and me as well (yes, I'm on the same journey).

Lockdown health is for anyone and everyone.

Don't think that generating creative ideas is something that is reserved only for some

health personalities like runners, walkers, dancer, swimmer, etc. Also, don't misunderstand that "Lockdown health" is only for those who want to put a dent in the world. Don't set yourself into some secluded category and limit yourself for a conventional path that delivers just results. Creative thinking is for anyone who wants to think and act differently from the standard way of doing things and thinking of different ways of arriving at best solutions by spending lesser time, money, and energy is and should be the objective of every health-oriented individual.

"Start with WHY" this Book is Authored by Simon Sinek. The author states that all the great leaders in the world inspire others by putting the Why (the purpose) before the How (the process), or the What (the product).

Big Take Away from the Book is

Your WHY is your purpose, cause, or belief.

Every inspiring leader and organization, regardless of size/industry, start with WHY

People don't buy WHAT you do, they buy WHY you do it.

Knowing our WHY is essential for lasting success.

When your WHY goes fuzzy, it becomes much more difficult to maintain the growth, loyalty, and inspiration that helped drive your original success.

Introduction: Key Takeaways

Even if you find limited alternatives to any problem, there are still more solutions to any problem.

Obesity Individuals and organizations equally can challenge their existing way of health and observe the things by shifting their perspective and approach of looking at any problem.

Yoga: The wellbeing, personal, as well as organization level examples, demonstrate that out of the box thinking opens up new paradigms and widens the perspective of looking at the world and out of box thinking is not uniquely gifted to some artistic profile people, nor is it limited to reality-bending world-changing successful entrepreneurs.

Meditation helps in the overall well being of your health and mind.

You are your coach. Anyone can develop their creative thinking faculties and generate surprisingly new and unpredictable ways of solving problems if they believe so and are willing to spend time in health and effort in learning how to do think out of the box.

Workouts types to Improve Health and Fitness Levels

Abdomen workout: Getting in shape through abdomen workout daily or alternate day to maintain the waist or obesity.

Running: Help to build strong bones, as it is a weight-bearing exercise, strengthen muscles, improve cardiovascular fitness, burn plenty of calories, help maintain a healthy weight.

Walking: Walking wards off heart disease, brings up the heart rate, lowers blood pressure and strengthens the heart., improve Circulation., increases the strength of your Bones and muscles, enjoy a longer Life, Lighten Your Mood, lose Weight and improve Sleep.

Dance: Dance health benefits are improved condition of your heart and lungs, increased muscular strength, increased aerobic fitness, improved muscle tone and strength, weight management or lose weight, stronger bones and reduced risk of osteoporosis, better coordination, agility, and flexibility.

Swimming: Swimming is an individual or team racing sport or good all-round activity that requires the use of one's entire body to move through water because it: keeps your heart rate up but takes some of the impact stress off your body, muscle strength, and cardiovascular fitness helps maintain a healthy weight, healthy heart, and lungs.

Cycling: "You are likely to fall if you stop paddling. As long as you don't give up in life, you will never end up failing"

Weight loss tips: Eat a high protein breakfast, avoid sugary drinks and fruit juice, drink water before meals, choose weight-loss-friendly foods, soups, use smaller plates, less sugar, intermittent fasting, good sleep, eat vegetables, drink coffee or green tea, eat slowly.

Massage improves our health and removes illness.

Smoking and the affects of smoking to various organs.

The **joy of giving** helps in improving one's mental health and health.

This book is a roadmap to learning and implementing the strategies for every health growth-oriented individual who want to explore and lead their life in a way that they couldn't have comprehended earlier.

Conclusion

May I ask you for a small favor?

CHAPTER 1

Introduction

"If you fail, never give up because FAIL means First Attempt In Learning."

...Dr. APJ Abdul Kalam

Health is a state of complete physical, mental, and social well-being and not merely the absence of disease. (WHO) or the condition where the body is devoid of any abnormality.

Wellness is the act of practicing healthy habits on a regular daily basis to attain better physical and mental health outcomes.

A gym is a club, or a room, usually containing special equipment, where people go to do physical exercise and get become fit. The gym is the activity of doing physical exercises in a gym, especially at school, college, or in the office.

Exercise is the physical action, which enhances the strength of the body, when performed in the required amount.

Feature of proper exercise is sweating, increased respiration rate, tightness in the body, and increased heartbeat.

The benefits of exercise are the lightness of the body, the ability to work, less fatigue etc.

Exercise nourishes the body, gives good complexion, takes away laziness, purifies the body, enhances tolerance power to tiredness, heat, and cold, increases life span and strength, and also gives good health.

"Fitness" is it refers to your optimal health and overall well-being of a person. Being fit not only means physical health but emotional, social well being, and mental health.

You should work out every day and doing some form of physical activity each day is smart when you're trying to slim down. But if you want to lose weight, repeating the same workout mode, intensity, or duration day but doing different will work.

CHAPTER 2

Obesity

"You cannot change your future, but you can change your habits, and surely your habits will change your future."

...Dr. APJ Abdul Kalam

What is Obesity? What Are the Causes? What is the Management/Prevention of Obesity?

The worldwide prevalence of obesity has doubled since1980.

Obesity is defined as the obese persons are deficient in longevity, slow in movement, difficulty in sexual intercourse, weakness, excessive sweating, excessive hunger, and thirst.

The prevalence of obesity in India is increasing and ranges from 8% to 38% in rural and 13% to 50% in urban areas obesity is more commonly seen in women compared to men and is increasing in children and adolescents. The state of Punjab (North India) has the highest prevalence of 30% in women and 22% in men and other cities are following this trend. Obesity has serious implications because it is associated with a two fold risk in heart disease and diabetes and an increased incidence in upper respiratory problems, and other health problems. Coming to Malaysia in the past decade, various steps have been taken to reduce this obesity. Among the steps taken was the '10,000 steps a day' campaign in 2009 by the Malaysian Ministry of Health. 'My Health' program was also launched by the Malaysian Health Promotion Board to increase nutrition by encouraging healthy food choices and weight reduction.

Definition of childhood obesity. Although the definition of obesity and overweight can be defined as an excess of Body Fat (BF). The Malaysian Ministry of Education also initiated the '1S 1S' (One student, One Sports) program intending to get more school children to become more physically active. All these programs have good objective and are supposed to reduce the prevalence of obesity in Malaysia. Children have been deprived of regular physical activity in their daily lives and studies reported that there were some beneficial effects of lifestyle intervention among the obese children and physical activity during physical education classes were at its minimum level in many schools as physical education is not monitored. The danger of adult obesity was greater for children who were at higher levels of obesity and for children who were obese at older ages.

Childhood obesity has reached epidemic levels in developed as well as in developing countries, and overweight, and obesity in childhood are known to have an effect on both physical and psychological health. Obese children are likely to stay obese into adulthood and develop non-communicable diseases like diabetes and cardiovascular diseases at a younger age. Environmental factors and lifestyle play crucial roles in the rising prevalence of obesity worldwide. In general, overweight and obesity are the results of an increase in caloric and fat intake and on the other hand, there are supporting evidence that excessive sugar, increased food intake, and less physical activity have been playing major roles in the rising obesity all around the world. Childhood obesity can highly affect children's physical health, social and mental well-being, and self-esteem. There is 50% of the adults are overweight and obese in many countries, it is difficult to reduce excessive weight once it becomes confirmed. The world is undergoing a rapid epidemiological and nutritional transition characterized by nutritional deficiencies, as evidenced by the prevalence of anemia, and iron and zinc deficiencies. There is a rise in the prevalence of obesity, diabetes, and other nutrition-related chronic diseases like obesity, diabetes, cardiovascular disease, hypertension, abnormal glucose tolerance, infertility and some forms of cancer.

Cause of obesity: obesity occurs when energy intake exceeds energy expenditure. There are multiple etiologies for this imbalance. Genetic factors influence the susceptibility of a given child to an obesity-conducive environment and environmental factors, lifestyle, and cultural environment seem to play major roles in the rising prevalence of obesity worldwide.

Studies have shown that actions like watching television and playing computer games are associated with obesity and during lockdown more free time results in less physical activity. Parents report that they prefer having their children watch television at home rather than play outside on its own during lockdown because parents are then able to complete their housework keeping an eye on their children. Increased children who are being driven to school and low participation rates in sports and physical education, particularly among adolescent girls, are also associated with increased obesity.

Prevention: Almost all health researchers and clinicians agree that prevention could be the key strategy and treatment for controlling the current epidemic of obesity during childhood. Prevention may include primary prevention of overweight or obesity, secondary prevention or avoidance of weight recovers following weight loss. It involves the walking on footpaths, the cycling network like roads, public open spaces (parks). The local environment, both school, and the wider community play an important role in shaping children's physical activity, the home environment are important in shaping children's eating behaviors and physical activity. Recent efforts in preventing obesity include the initiative of using school report cards to make the parents aware of their children's weight problem and Health report cards are believed to support in prevention of obesity.

Conclusion: During lockdown, overweight and obesity in childhood have a significant impact on both physical and psychological health and psychological disorders such as depression occur with increased frequency in obese children. Overweight children are more likely to have cardiovascular in adulthood as compared with those who are thin. These strategies can be initiated at home and in school, college, etc influencing the diet and physical activity at home and work for adults. We offer some specific traditional Indian customs which may offer innovative solutions like yoga.

CHAPTER 3

Yoga

"Good health is not something we can buy. However, it can be an extremely valuable savings account."

...Anne Wilson Schaef

Which Yoga Asanas to Help You Burn Belly Fat?

Yoga during lockdown/or any other time if encouraged can help in preventing stress and may well turn out to be a low-cost strategy in preventing diabetes, obesity, and cardiovascular disease. However, the implementation of yoga should take place in the schools and colleges of India/world

1. Naukasana. (Fig 1)

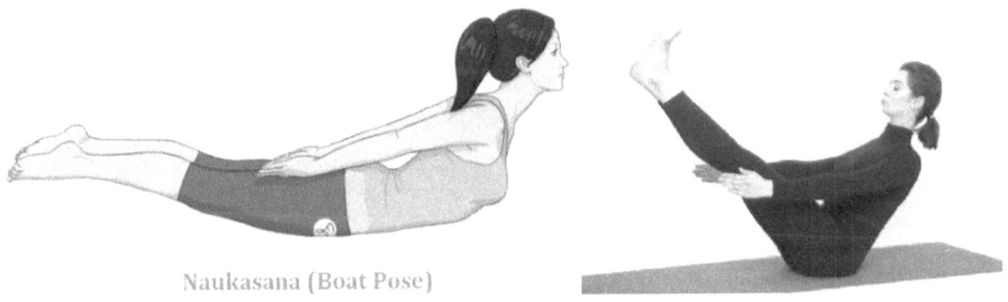

Naukasana (Boat Pose)

Nauka means boat, Asana is a posture and here the shape of the boat is formed.

A Step-by-Step Guide to Do Naukasana

1. First lie down flat on yoga mat, with feet together and arms on the sides.

2. Keep arms straight and fingers outstretched towards your toes.

3. Start inhaling and as you exhale, lift chest and feet off the ground, stretching your arms towards feet. Feel the tightness in stomach area as the abdominal muscles contract.

4. Let the weight of body rest on the buttocks. Make sure eyes, finger, and toes are all in one line. Hold breath and remain in this position for a few seconds.

5. Exhale slowly as you bring the body down to the starting position and relax. Perform 3–4 repetitions daily.

Benefits

1. Naukasana strengthens the abdominal muscles.

2. Nauksana helps improve and regulate your digestion, including alleviating excessive gas and easing constipation.

3. The stretching, compressing, and relaxation of the abdominal region involved with asana is a really good for burning belly fat if practiced regularly.

4. It strengthen the muscles of the neck, shoulder, and legs.

5. Contraindicated in patients with Asthma and heart patients.

2. Vajrasana or diamond pose. (Fig 2)

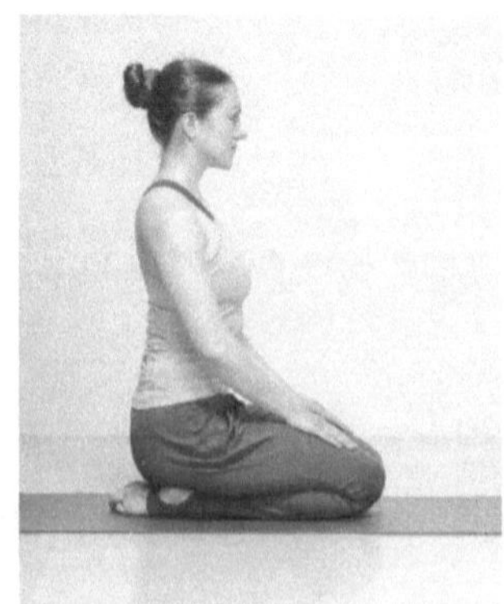

Vajra means Diamond. Normally Asanas should perform on an empty stomach. Here, Vajrasana can be done immediately after the meal and helps in proper digestion. Tighten the thigh like the diamond and knees.

Steps

1. Sit erect with legs straight.

2. The head should face the sky and head should be straight, facing forward.

3. Place your hands on knees and start by breathing and exhaling slowly.

4. Make sure to watch your breath and close your eyes when you.

5. Breathe in and out at a natural pace for five to ten minutes.

Benefits

1. Improves Digestion: Vajrasana (the thunderbolt pose) is known to improve digestion and and helps to prevent stomach ulcers, eliminate constipation.

2. Loosens Up Your Back Muscles: If you spend time at a desk all day during lockdown, you'll find that the Vajrasana procedure is perfect for loosening up back muscles. It will strengthen the muscles in your spine, and eliminate back pain.

3. Helps You To Meditate: It's one of the few asanas that make meditation a lot easier as you breathe in and out deeply.

4. Improve Blood Circulation: The Vajrasana position helps in blood circulation throughout your body that is this makes legs and arms warm up and move around more easily.

5. Prevents Obesity: Vajrasana helps in metabolism and keeps you in great shape. Since this is a relaxing pose and helps to eliminate cravings and overeating after meals.

3. Pavanamukthasana (Fig 3)

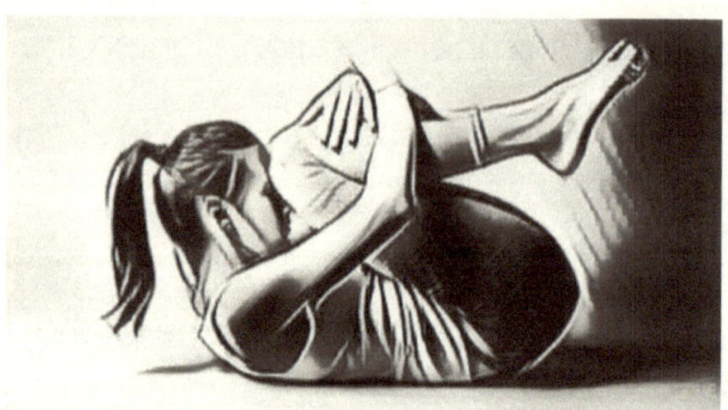

Pawan – wind, Mukta – relieve or release, Asana – pose.

The Wind-Relieving Pose (Pawanmuktasana) is a lie down posture that is suitable for everyone, whether they are beginners or advanced.

This yoga must be practiced at least four to six hours after a meal when stomach is empty.

Steps To Do Pawanmuktasana

1. Lie flat on your back on a smooth surface, ensuring that your feet are together and arms are placed beside your body.

2. Take a deep breath. As you exhale, bring knees towards your chest, and press thighs on your abdomen. Hold your hands around your legs as if you are hugging your knees.

3. Hold the asana while you breathe normally. Every time you exhale, make sure you tighten the grip of the hands-on the upper shins and increase the pressure on chest. Every time you inhale, you loosen the grip.

4. Exhale and release the pose after you rock and roll from side to side about three to six times. Relax

Benefits

1. It strengthens the abdominal muscles and internal organs of the digestive system, therefore improving digestion.

2. It strengthens the back muscles and tones the muscles of the arms and the legs.

3. It improves the circulation of blood.

4. It stimulates the reproductive organs and massages the pelvic muscles.

5. It aids in burning fat in the thighs, buttocks, and abdominal area.

4. Paschimottanasana (Seated Forward Bend) Paschim: — west, back, back of body‖ uttana: —intense stretch, straight, extended‖ āsana: —posture (Fig 4)

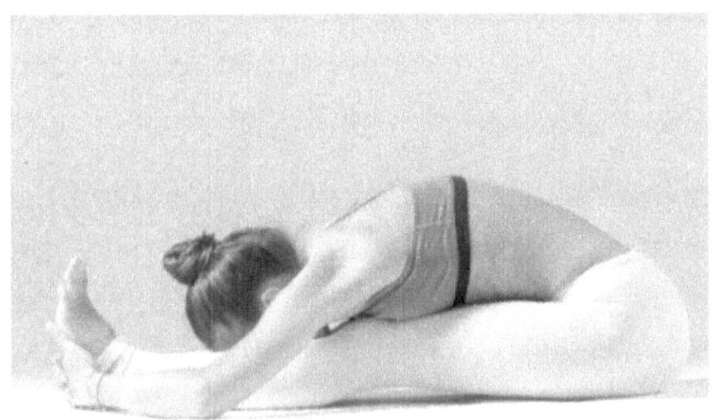

Steps to do Paschimottanasana

Begin by coming to sit in Dandasana with legs straight in front of your body

1. Bring arms to the sides and up over your head, reaching toward the ceiling.

2. Inhale and draw spine up long.

3. As you exhale, begin to come forward, swinging your hips.

4. On each inhale, lengthen spine and you come out of your forward bend to do this.

5. On each exhale, deepen into your forward bend. Imagine belly coming to rest on your thighs, rather than nose coming to your knees and this will help keep your spine long.

6. Keep the neck as the natural extension of spine.

7. As you come to your full extension with the spine long, decide whether you want to stay here or let spine round forward.

8. Release the hands. Keep your feet flexed strongly throughout.

Benefits

1. Pashcimottanasana engages the body to achieve the final yoga pose. This asana stretches the spine, shoulders, thighs, and calf muscles thereby allowing your body an excellent stretch..

2. One of the best health benefits of Paschimottanasana is that it relieves the mental and physical stress thereby calming the body and mind. Paschimottanasana rejuvenates the overall well being with its well-formed yoga pose.

3. The common problem faced by the people today is excess belly fat and the natural remedy to curb such unwanted belly fat by Paschimottanasana. Practicing Paschimottanasana involves abdominal stretch which reduces the excess abdominal fat and tones the body beautifully.

4. Hatha yoga with its yoga asanas massages and tones the abdominal and pelvic organs which heals the body from different abdominal disorders like ulcerative colitis, gastric issues, pancreatitis. The yoga asana heavily benefits the women at the time of menstruation by softening the menstrual cramps and toning the abdominal organs. Furthermore, there are excellent benefits of Paschimottanasana are this yoga pose is beneficial for the ovaries, uterus, kidneys, and liver. The seated forward bend pose helps at the

time of menopause and prevents episodes at the time of pregnancy.

5. Paschimottanasana benefits by stimulating the proper functioning of the digestive organs. Improved digestion leads to proper absorption of food which gives a healthy body.

6. Another top benefit of Paschimottanasana is that a regular practice of this hatha yoga asana improves wellbeing and improves the body's energy thereby removing the body weakness. Paschimottanansana reduces fatigue, and strength to the daily lifestyle.

7. Seated Forward Bend helps one to land on an upright posture to reach the state of Meditation. A peaceful state of mind is conducive to meditation. Paschimottanasana gives a relaxation to the mind and soul leading you towards ultimate wellbeing and spirituality.

5. Padahastasana (Fig 5)

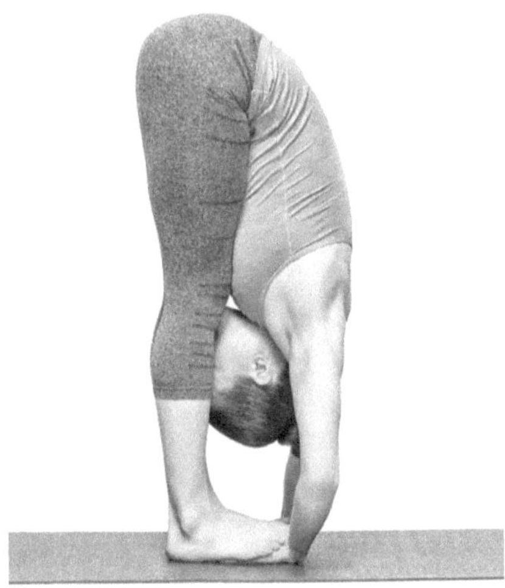

'Pada' means foot, Hasta means hands and this posture is keeping palm next to the foot.

Steps

1. Distance your legs hip-width apart.

2. Inhale and slowly raise arms upwards and stretch your body upwards as well.

3. Exhale and slowly bend the trunk forward from your hips till hands reach your feet.

4. Next, place the palms of hands under the soles.

5. Elbows remain slightly bent pointing outwards.

Stay in this position for as long as you feel comfortable.

Practice the pose 3 times for 5 breaths gradually increasing the time day by day as your flexibility increases.

Benefits

1. Eliminates stress, anxiety, and fatigue by energizing the body.

2. Padahastasana improves balance, posture, and flexibility.

3. Improves blood circulation in the upper part of the body.

4. Beneficial for people suffering from problems related to throat and nasal.

5. Increases concentration and speeds up metabolism.

6. Beneficial for people suffering from gastric problems, abdominal bloating, and indigestion.

Precautions for Padahastasana (Hand under foot pose)

1. People suffering from severe back pain, high blood pressure, heart problems, knee problems, or abdominal hernia.

2. Overstretching might put a lot of stress on knees, thigh, calf, ankle, and may result in a sprain.

3. Don't strain the body. Practice according to capability and flexibility.

6. Trikonasana (Fig 6)

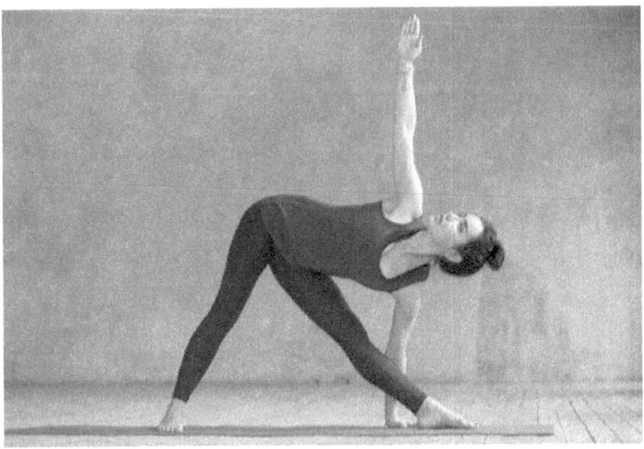

'Trikona' means triangle. This posture forms a triangle with extended arms and feet.

Steps

Yoga beginners always do a good warm-up exercise of the whole body before doing this asana.

1. Stand erect and then spread the legs apart with 2 ½ to 3 feet gap.

2. Raise the arm and position them parallel to the ground.

3. Then the right foot 90^0 to the right, bend the trunk to the right side with an exhalation, place the right palm next to the right foot.

4. Keep both the arms in a straight line and look towards the thumb of the left hand.

5. Maintain this posture for some time with normal breathing and the same procedure should be repeated on the left side.

Benefits of Trikonasana (Triangle Pose)

1. Trikonasana helps to strengthen your legs, ankles, and knees.

2. Trikonasana is good for your digestion

3. Trikonasana pose helps to expand your chest and shoulders.

4. Trikonasana, it provides stamina, balance, energy, and develops focus.

5. Trikonasana helps to strengthen the muscles in the hips, thighs, and back.

6. Trikonasana is done in conditions of weight and obesity because this asana is good to burn fat.

7. Trikonasana helps to improve balance and increase concentration.

8. Trikonasana, reduces anxiety, stress, back pain.

Precaution to do Trikonasana

a) If you are suffering from back and spinal injuries.

b) Person with high or low blood pressure patients.

c) Person who is suffering from Migraine.

d) Person, who is suffering from diarrhea, neck, and back injuries.

e) If you are performing this asana, then don't take the support of knee as it exerts excess pressure on your knee that may lead to knee problems.

f) Especially for pregnant women if there is any complication, then you should practice under the expert guidance and consult a doctor before performing Trikonasana.

7. Adho Mukha Svanasana (Fig 7)

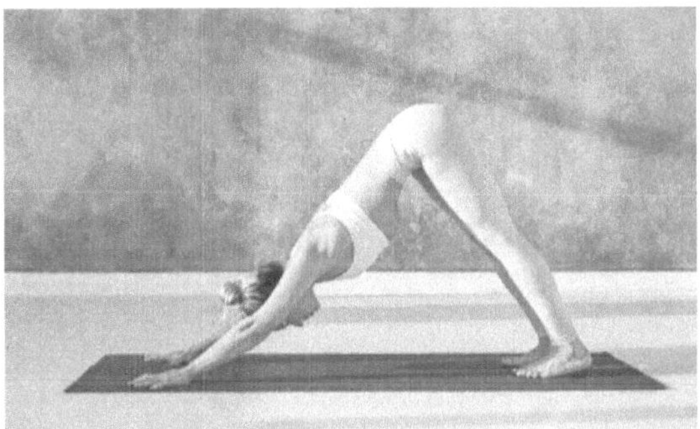

Steps

1. Come onto the floor on hands and knees. Set your knees directly below your hips and your hands slightly forward of your shoulders and spread palms, index fingers parallel or slightly turned out, and turn your toes under.

2. Exhale and lift your knees away from the floor. At first, keep the knees slightly bent and the heels lifted away from the floor and lengthen your tailbone away from the back of your pelvis and press it lightly. Against this resistance, lift the sitting bones toward the ceiling, and from inner ankles draw the inner legs up into the groins.

3. Then with an exhalation, push your top thighs back and stretch heels onto or down toward the floor. Straighten your knees. Firm the outer thighs and roll the upper thighs inward slightly. Narrow the front of the pelvis.

4. Firm the outer arms and press the bases of the index fingers actively into the floor. From these two points lift along your inner arms from the wrists to the tops of the shoulders. Firm your shoulder blades against your back, then widen them and draw them toward the tailbone. Keep the head between the upper arms.

5. It's also an excellent yoga asana all on its own. Stay in this pose anywhere from 1 to 3 minutes. Then bend your knees to the floor with an exhalation and rest.

Benefits

1. Calms the brain and helps relieve stress and depression.

2. Energizes the body.

3. Stretches the shoulders, hamstrings, calves, arches, and hands.

4. Strengthens the arms and legs.

5. Helps relieve the symptoms of menopause.

6. Relieves menstrual discomfort when done with head supported.

7. Helps prevent osteoporosis.

8. Improves digestion.

9. Relieves headache, back pain, and fatigue.

Pregnancy: This pose should be avoided in late-trimester

8. Uttanpadasana (Raised Foot Pose). **(Fig 8)**

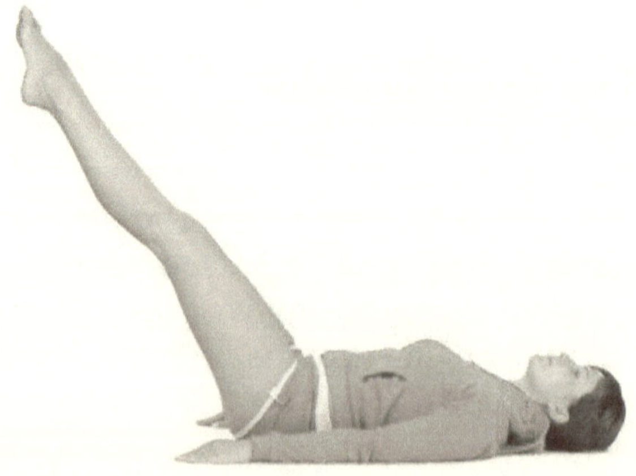

In Sanskrit Uttan means Raised, Pad means Leg and Asana means Pose, so the combination of all the words, it's pronounced as The Raised Leg Pose beside this while doing Uttanpadasana legs are lifted in the air.

Steps to do Uttanpadasana (The Raised Leg Pose):

1. To start this asana lie flat on your back on your yoga mat, breathe normally. Both your hands should be placed alongside your body and your palm should be facing down a word.

2. Now inhale slowly and try to lift your leg from the floor and keep your leg at a 45 – 60-degree angle from the floor.

3. Your upper body should be parallel to the floor and try to keep your leg straight.

4. Hold in this position for some time at least for 15 to 20 seconds to feel pressure in lower abs.

5. Beginners, try to be in this position for 2 to 3 breaths.

6. To release from this position, breathe out and slowly lower legs to the floor. Now keep both hands alongside your body, keep leg straight and take a deep breath and relax.

7. Now again do this asana. You should do a minimum of 10 repetitions of this asana for better results.

8. Initially, when you start this yogasana, you feel some pain in your abdomen, hip, thigh, but as you practice more you can do this asana more easily.

Benefits

1. Prevents Acidity, Indigestion, and Constipation, Cures Back Pain,

2. Strengthens the Abdominal Organs,

3.   Improve the Function of Reproductive Organs,

4.   Improve the Function of Digestive Systems.

5.   Strengthens the Back, Hip, and Thigh Muscles.

Contraindicated

1.   In people who are suffering from a severe back injury, abdomen pain, and recently any surgery on your back or waist, spinal column disease on the lower vertebrae they should not do this asana.

2.   Those who are suffering from high or low blood pressure, they should not do this asana without any supervision.

3.   For women, those who were Pregnant should avoid Uttanpadasana for the first few months, but they can do this asana by consulting with the doctor from the third trimester and women should not practice in days of periods.

9. Ashwasan— (Fig 9)

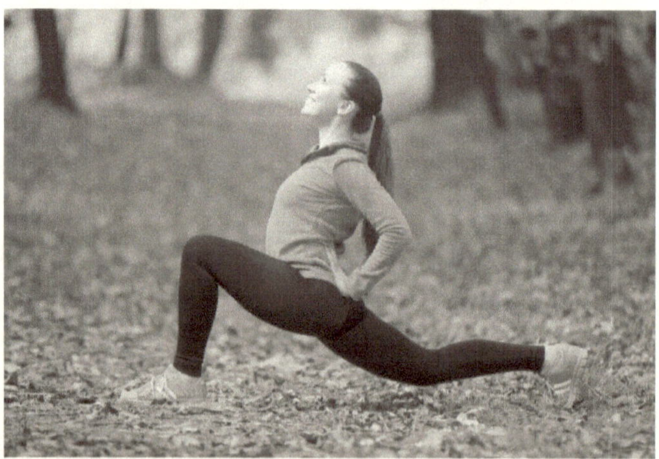

In Sanskrit, Ashwa means the Horse. After putting in hard labor for the whole day, the horse gets rid of all his tiredness and gets energy in just a few minutes, simply by moving its legs in one direction and the head and the neck in the other direction and thus he is again ready for work. That is why this posture/asana is called The Horse Posture/Ashwasan

Steps to do Ashwa Asana

1. Lie on a mat, facing upwards. Bend both the legs at the knees, join the feet and the knees of both the legs, and spread the arms at the right angle to your body. Forms fists with hands the keep these fists under your head.

2. While breathing in, rotate knees to the left side and move head to the right side so that the chin touches the right shoulder. The feet are to be kept placed together.

3. Now, twist your body as you twist the towel to squeeze it dry. Then come to the normal position while breathing out. Now, breathing in again, rotate knees and head in the opposite direction.

4. Breathe in while practicing this posture and breathe out while this posture is nearing completion. Rotating the knees to the left and then to the right, forms one complete set of this posture. Practice five to ten such sets. This posture can also be practiced while keeping a gap of 18 to 20 cms between the feet.

Benefits of Ashwa Asana

1. People suffering from constipation should practice this posture 25 to 50 minutes after drinking naturally cold or warm water. They will find relief in constipation. If this posture is practiced when one is feeling lazy, then one feels energetic.

2. If this posture is practiced before going to bed, then one gets deep sleep.

3. As the age of person advances, a person gets a hunch back (bent back) and one can delay the onset of old age

by performing this posture. Even the bent back becomes straight again.

4. Complaints of the backbone, back, slipped disc, spondylitis, etc are diminished with the help of this posture.

10. Dhanurasana (Fig 10)

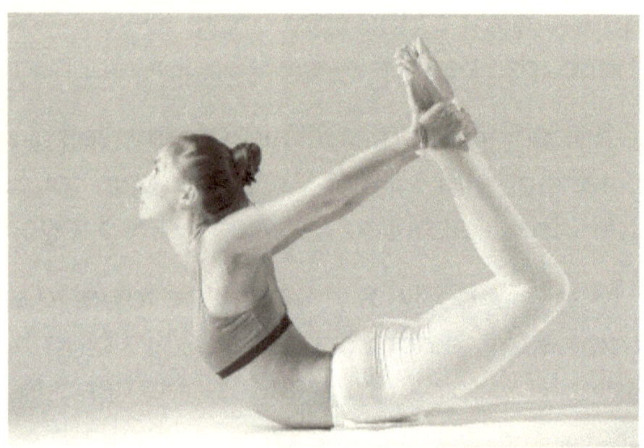

Steps

1. To do this posture, first lie down on the stomach.

2. Now while exhaling, bring the knees close to the waist and hold both ankles with your hand.

3. While breathing, raise your head, chest, and thigh upwards as much as possible, lift the body upward.

4. During this time try to take the weight of your body on the lower abdomen.

5. When you lift body completely, try to reduce the gap between the legs.

6. While doing this asana, the flow of your breath should be relaxed, breathe slowly, and exhale slowly.

7. After remaining in this position for about 15–20 seconds, return to the previous position while exhaling.

8. You can do this asana three to five times according to your benefit and ability.

Benefits of Dhanurasana – Bow Pose

1. Effective in weight loss.

2. Improves digestion and appetite.

3. Helps to cure obesity, rheumatism, and gastrointestinal problems.

4. Cures constipation.

5. Improves blood circulation.

6. Gives flexibility to the back and strengthens back muscles.

7. Improve the function of the liver, small intestine, and big intestine.

8. Act as a stress reliever.

9. Strengthens ankles, thighs, chest, and abdominal organs.

10. Cure menstruation disorder.

11. Improve the function of the kidney and liver.

12. It improves posture..

13. Cures respiratory disorders like asthma.

14. Helpful is stimulating reproductive organs.

15. Improve the function of the pancreas and it is beneficial in diabetes.

Precautions while doing Dhanurasana(bow pose)

1. Patients with heart diseases should avoid doing this asana. You may have problems due to stress on the heart.

2. People suffering from high blood pressure.

3. If you are suffering from hernia, ulcers, colitis, and any stomach disease, do not do this asana because this posture puts the maximum pressure on the stomach.

4. Do not do this asana for at least two-three hours after eating a meal.

5. Pregnant women should not perform Dhanurasana under any condition

11. Urdhva Mukha Shvanasana. (urdhva mukha = face upward (urdhva = upwardmukha = face) svana = dog **(Fig 11)**

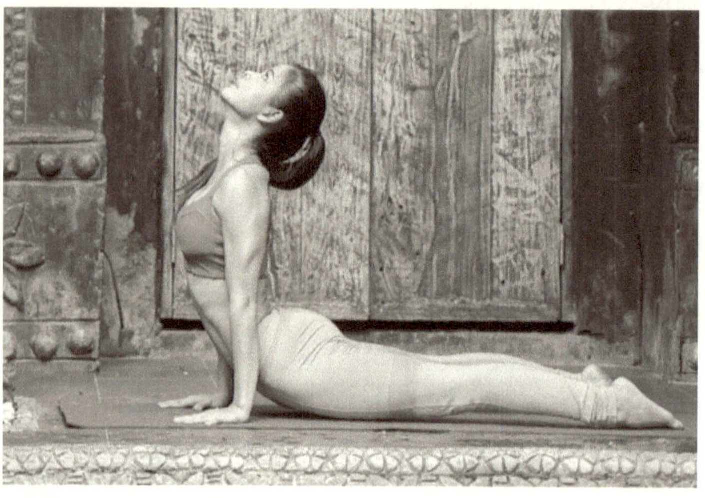

Upward-Facing Dog Pose

Step 1: Lie on the floor. Stretch your legs back, with the tops of feet on the floor. Bend elbows and spread your palms on the floor beside waist so that forearms are relatively perpendicular to the floor.

Step 2: Inhale and press inner hands firmly into the floor and slightly back, as if you were trying to push yourself forward along the floor. Then straighten your arms and simultaneously lift your torso and legs a few inches off the floor on an inhalation. Keep the thighs firm and slightly turned inward, the arms firm and turned out so the elbow creases face forward.

Step 3: Press the tailbone toward the pubis and lift the pubis toward the navel. Narrow the hip points. Firm but don't harden the buttocks.

Step 4: Firm the shoulder blades against the back and puff the side ribs forward. Lift through the top of the sternum but avoid pushing the front ribs forward. Look straight ahead or tip the head back slightly, but take care not to compress the back of the neck.

Step 5: Urdhva Mukha Svanasana is one of the positions in the traditional Sun Salutation sequence. You can also practice this pose individually, holding it anywhere from 15 to 30 seconds, breathing easily. Release back to the floor or lift into Adho Mukha Svanasana with an exhalation.

Benefits

1. Improves posture.

2. Strengthens the spine, arms, wrists.

3. Stretches chest and lungs, shoulders, and abdomen.

4. Firms the buttocks.

5. Stimulates abdominal organs.

6. Helps relieve mild depression and fatigue.

7. Good for a patient with asthma.

Contraindications

1. Back injury.

2. Headache.

3. Pregnancy

12. Balasana:

In Sanskrit, Bala means child, and asana refers to one's posture. Thus, this pose is also called Child Pose.

Steps To Do Balasana yoga (Child Pose)

1. To do Balasan, place a Yoga mat in an open area. Sit on your knees on the yoga mats that are Vajrasana. In this case, rest your upper body on the thighs. (Fig 12)

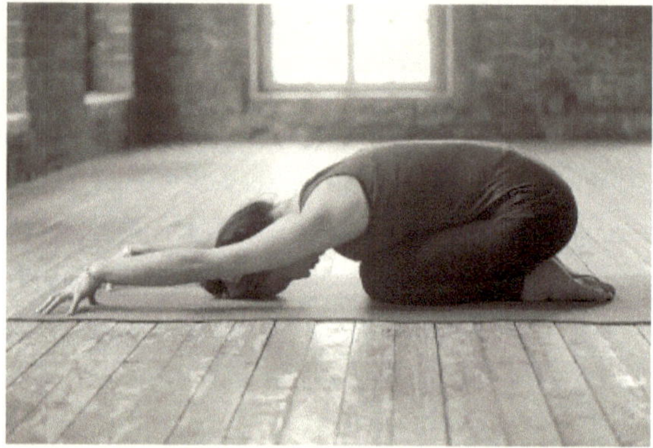

2. Keep both knees of your feet sticking to each other or at a short distance from each other and keep the waist perfectly straight and now take a deep breath and tilt the upper body towards the front. Keep both hands backward and note that your palms keep touching the body. And try that the head touches the ground in front.

3. After coming in this posture, slowly bring your chest by pressing towards the thighs and chest should touch both thighs. Try to pull the tailbone towards the pelvis. After this, remove the hands from both sides of the body and keep it on the ground while extending forward, palms placed facing down on the mat.

4. If it is not comfortable, then you keep the forehead relaxed by placing the other palm on top of one palm and keep your

breath normal, this condition is called Balasana. Remain in this posture for 1 minute and keep breathing slowly.

To get out of this easy, first, bring your palms under the shoulder and slowly raise your upper body and return to the previous position and breathe.

Benefits of Balasana

1. Helps relieve fatigue and resting pose, it helps relax the body.

2. This is also a great pose to ease anxiety and stress and breathing helps relax the mind.

3. It also gently stretches the ankles, hips, and shoulders.

4. Stimulates digestion and elimination.

5. It helps ease neck and back pain.

Balasana Contraindications

1. Should be avoided by pregnant women.

2. Knee injury.

3. Infection in the stomach.

4. Severe spondylitis.

5. Injury at the ankle.

13. Bhujangasana (Cobra Pose) (Fig 13)

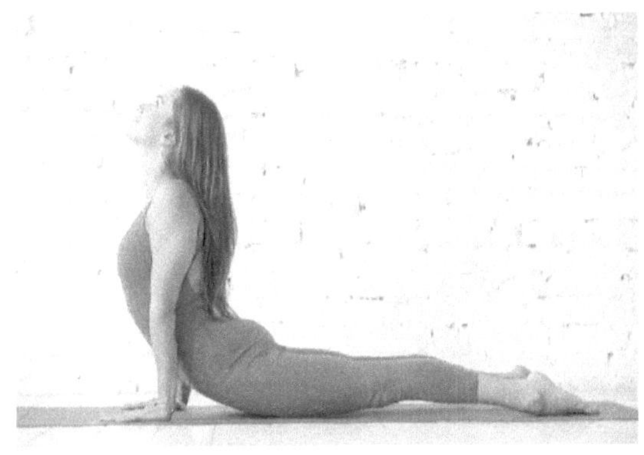

1. Lie flat on your stomach keeping your legs straight, feet together, heels slightly touching each other and toes pointing

2. Rest the palm of your hands by the side of chest, your arms must be close to body with elbows pointing outward.

3. Rest your forehead on the floor and relax your body.

4. Inhale and raise your forehead, neck, and then shoulders. Using your back muscles raise your chest, now use the strength of your arms to raise your trunk. Look upward breathing normally. This is the final position.

5. In the final position, your navel should not raise more than 3cm; with pubic bones touching the floor. Hold this position for 20–25 seconds.

6. To come back to the starting position first exhale and then slowly lower your navel, chest, shoulders, neck, and forehead. Relax and take deep breaths.

Bhujangasana (Cobra Pose) Benefits

Being the 7th posture of Suryanamaskar, it has several benefits such as:

1. Strengthens the spine, keeps it strong, healthy, and flexible.

2. Gives a good stretch to neck, shoulder, chest, lungs, and abdomen.

3. Helps in the functioning of abdominal organs such as kidney and liver.

4. Beneficial in menstrual and other disorders of the female reproductive system.

5. Useful for people suffering from back pain, slipped disc, and cervical spondylitis.

6. Relieves stress and anxiety and calms the mind.

Practice this asana 3–5 times, before or after a forward bending pose such as Paschimottanasana

(seated forward bend) will give you maximum benefits. With regular practice, you will be able to straighten your arms, the spine to a greater extent.

Precautions for Bhujangasana (Cobra Pose)

1. Some people are naturally flexible while some are not and a lot of us have very stiff muscles and give your body the time it needs to gain strength and flexibility.

2. Take very little support of arms, use back muscles to hold the weight of your upper body in the pose that is how your spine is going to get stronger.

3. Your feet might raise a bit from the ground unintentionally, try to keep them down.

4. Practice this asana under the guidance of an instructor if you suffer from any of this condition: hyperthyroidism, hernia, peptic ulcer.

14. Surya Namaskara – (Fig 14) It is combination of different asana

Step (Asana)	Mantra (name of Surya)	Translation
Tadasana	Om Mitraya Namah	Affectionate to all
Urdhva Hastasana	Om Ravaye Namah	cause of all changes
Padahastasana	Om Sūryāya Namah	Who induces all activity
Ashwa Sanchalanasana	Om Bhānave Namah	Who diffuses light

Continued...

Parvatasana	Om Khagāya Namah	who moves in the sky
Ashtanga Namaskara	Om Pusne Namah	Who nourishes all
Bhujangasana	Om Hiraya Garbhāya Namah	Who contains everything
Parvatasana	Om Mariaye Namah	Who possesses raga

Steps

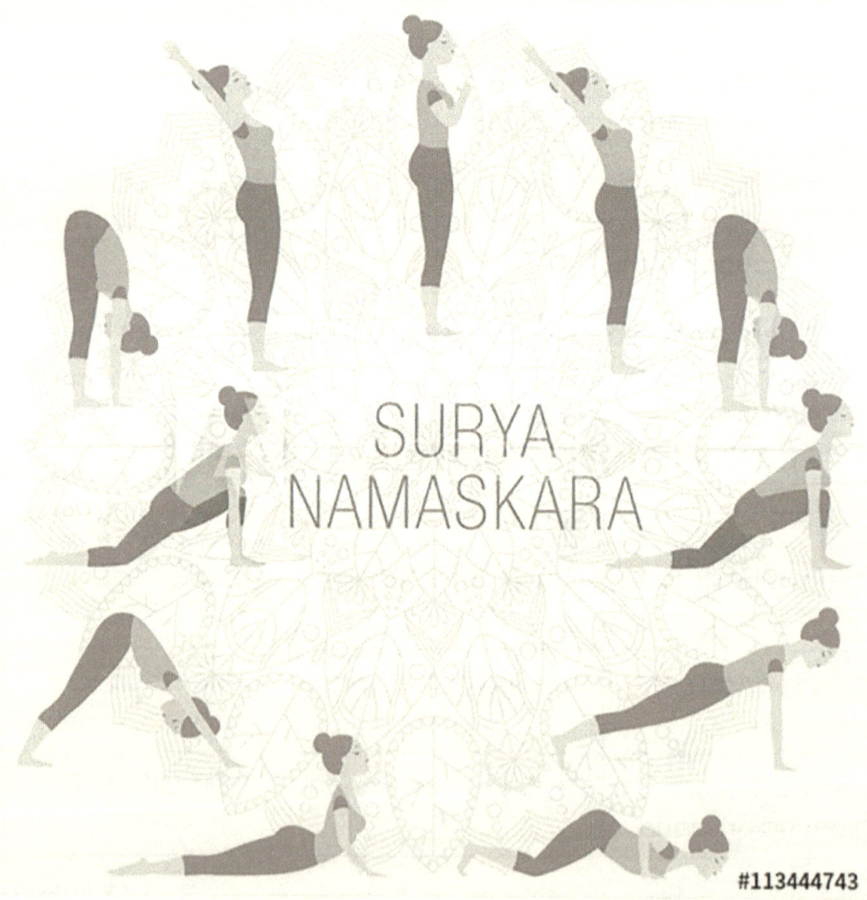

Position 1

Prarthanasan: Both feet touching each other, both hands are joined at the center of the chest as in prayer position back and neck straight and look straight.

Breathing: Kumbhak

Benefit: Helps to keep the balance of the body.

Position 2

Continuing from the first position take hands straight up above your head and bend slightly backward to stretch your back. Keep your hands in a prayer position (without bending your elbows). Keep your neck between your arms and looking upwards bend slightly backward from the waist.

Breathing: Purak (From going from Position 1 to 2 slowly, start taking long breaths) Benefit: Strengthens chest muscles which in turn help in breathing.

Position 3

Uttanasan: Maintaining from 2nd position take your hands from above your head bending in the front and place your hands beside your feet on both sides. Keep your knees straight and try to touch the head to your knees.

Breathing: Rechak (Leave your breath slowly while you go from Position 2 to 3)

Benefit: Makes the waist and spine flexible. It strengthens the muscles and is beneficial for the functioning of the liver.

Position 4

Ekpad prasarnasan: From the 3rd position start sitting down and take one leg backward in full stretching position, your hands resting on the ground on either side of the front leg. The other leg should be bent at the knee put the chest weight on the front knee, your eyes should be looking upwards.

Breathing: Purak

Benefit: Strengthens the leg muscles and makes the spine and neck muscles flexible.

Position 5

Chaturang dandasan: Now slowly take the second leg behind and beside the first. Keep the legs in line with the knees. The whole body weight should rest on the palms and toes. The foot, waist, and head should be in a straight line and look in front towards the ground (This is also called Chaturang Dandasan because the body rests on the toes and palms)

Breathing: Rechak

Benefit: Strengthens the arms and keeps body posture

Position 6

Ashtangasan: Lower the chest down the ground bending both arms at the elbows. The following eight organs should touch the ground, forehead, chest, both palms, both knees, and both toes. (Because eight body parts touch the ground it is called Ashtangasan)

Breathing: Kumbhak (Bahirkumbak)

Benefit: Press the spine and waist flexible and strengthens the muscles.

Position 7

Bhujangasan: Now lift your body above the waist, bending it slightly backward and looking backward. Make sure legs and thighs are touching the ground and back is in a semi-circular position.

Breathing: Purak

Benefit: Makes the spine and waist flexible and strengthens the muscles. (Positions 5, 6, and 7 together, strengthen the arms and reduce the fat around the abdomen and waist.)

Position 8

Adhomukh svanasan: Lift your waist upwards and arms fully stretched with hands and legs resting on the ground, try to touch the chin to the chest.

Breathing: Rechak

Benefit: Beneficial for spine and waist muscles.

Position 9

Ekpad Prasarnasan: Same as the 4th position with the opposite leg behind.

Breathing: Purak

Position 10

Uttanasan: Same as that in the 3rd position.

Breathing: Rechak

Position 11 (Same as 2nd position)

Position 12 (same/coming back to position 1)

Prarthanasan: Both legs touching each other, both hands joined at the center of the chest as in prayer position back and neck straight and look straight.

—After that slowly come back to Position 1. Now one Surya Namaskar is over. Every day do at least twelve such Surya Namaskars.

Benefits of Surya Namaskar

A. It improves the blood circulation of all the important organs of the body.

B. Improves the functioning of the heart and lungs.

C. Strengthens the muscles of the arms and waist.

D. Makes the spine and waist more flexible.

E. Reduces the fat around the abdomen and thus reduces weight.

F. Improves digestion.

G. Improves concentration.

Contraindicated: In people with neck problems should consult a professional/yoga trainer before performing Surya namaskar

15. **Savasana: (Savasana means — Corpse Pose) Savasana is the final resting pose at the end of almost every yoga practice. (Fig 15)**

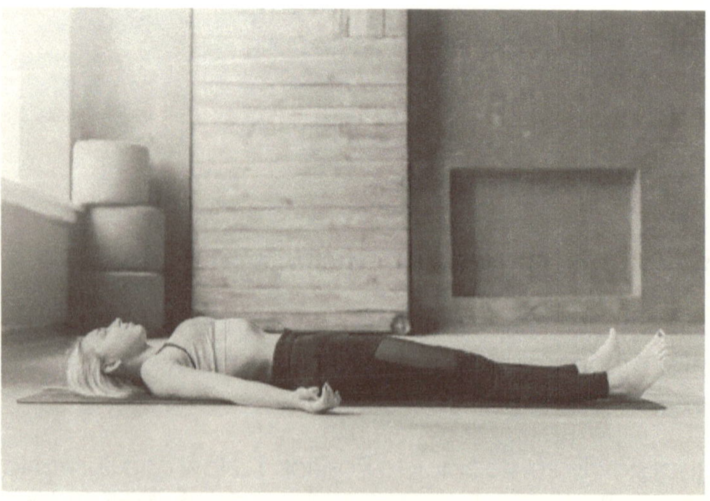

Steps

1. Lying down on the ground in the supine position like a dead body of savasana and stretch both legs.

2. The heels should be 12 to 20 inches apart and the feet should be at the sides with eyes and lips should be gently closed.

3. Take out-breath from the mouth and bring the stomach inward. Do this 3 times. Breathing should be normal.

Benefits

1. Soothing effect on the body.

2. Relaxes the body completely.

3. It is very useful for those who have high blood pressure. They should do it for 10 minutes in the morning and evening.

4. This Asana brings peace of mind and increases concentration, reduces the tension.

KARMA: In its most basic sense, the Law of Karma in the moral teaches that similar actions will lead to similar results so is the health. In physics, Sir Isaac Newton postulated that for every action there is an equal and opposite reaction. In metaphysics, karma is a law that states that every mental, emotional, and physical activity, no matter how insignificant is projected out into the psychic mind and eventually returns to the individual with equal impact. Phrases associated with karma law include – You Reap What You Sow or the – Fruits of Ones Labor. For example, I/ we plant a mango seed, the plant that springs up will be a mango tree, and eventually, it will bear a mango fruit. In the same way, if we plant a neem tree we can't get sweet mangoes. This says according to one's actions with the fruit. There is some belief that parents pass their karma to the children and some say karma is only individual. Since children inherit stuff from parents, some of their parent's bad karma will be passed down as well. Good karma always results in good health.

Karma-Yoga (Spirit at Work) is derived from Bhagavad Gita meaning to act without any concern for the outcome (Nishkama Karma). Karma-Yoga forms the basis of Indian work values and varies from the reformed work values in terms of the intention of the doer (karta) that is Indians consider work to be a duty, an duty towards others which one is indebted to them in a previous life, hence performing one's duty without desire for worldly gains will yield higher benefit like liberation (mukti) from the cycle of birth, death, and rebirth.

CHAPTER 4

Meditation

"A regular meditation practice is one of the highest forms of self-love."

...Renae. A. Sauter

Why to Do Meditation

Meditation is a practice where an individual uses a technique – such as directing the mind on a particular object, or activity. Meditation may be used to reduce stress, anxiety, depression, pain, and peace, perception, and well-being.

In Hinduism, Yoga and Dhyana are practiced to realize the union of one's soul. Just as we cannot see our image on a glass on which dust has settled, similarly, we cannot see the image of God when our heart is impure.

Mahatma Gandhi had said, —A man should first purify his heart. The best way to purify our heart is through prayer. When with a pure heart we pray to god, we get the strength to face difficulties.

Meditation & pranayama help us express ourselves better'

Sadhguru had said — Meditation means dissolving the invisible walls that unawareness has built.

How to Start Meditating/Prayer

The best time to pray is early morning. In the morning one should pray that he may be successful in his work during that day, and at night one should offer all his good work which he has done that day to God. He should pray for forgiveness if he has done anything wrong that day, and he should not repeat his mistakes. God has created everything. With prayer, we derive strength and this helps us to overcome all our problems and difficulties and make our journey in life successful.

Benefits of Meditation

- Reverse the stress

- Our heart rate and breathing slow down, our blood pressure normalizes, we use oxygen more efficiently and we sweat less.

- Mind ages at a slower rate.

8-minute meditation – a powerful and effective tool for lowering stress. 8 Minute Meditation is a natural, safe, and highly, safe, and highly effective — antidote to stress. A book, published in November 2005 by Victor Davich, this book is for someone who wants to get started with meditation instantly as meditation to be it perfect needs time and patience.

8 Minute Meditation Stress Reduction is designed to give the practitioner instant, simple, and powerful over stress.

To make prayer to God successful and effective we should observe the few conditions—

- a) Love for God

- b) Praise God.

- c) Remembering God

- d) Surrender to God.

- e) Meditation

- f) Purity of heart

- g) Observing silence

Procedure

1. Sit comfortable on chair or a mat.

2. Do lying down, if sitting to meditate is unappealing.

3. Put on the music of birds or slow instrumental or nature sounds, if that helps to calm you before beginning to meditate.

4. Set a digital (non-ticking) timer.

5. Breathe continuously your nose, with your mouth closed.

The world is turning to yoga for the numerous benefits this way of life offers. Yoga boosts your metabolism, improving your digestion. As the World Yoga Day celebrations, we leave you with five pranayamas that you must include in your daily life. Done frequently, they will help you beat stress, relax, calm your mind, and work.

1. ANULOM-VILOM

Also known as Nadi Shdodhana (alternate nostril breathing) You must do it at least 60 times, divided throughout the day. This is excellent for healing, chakra balancing, and getting rid of breathing or respiratory problems. This can be done even after meals.

What it does

This pranayama helps normalize blood pressure, aids in blood purification, reduced the risk of heart disease, and can also improve sight.

ANULOM-VILOM pranayama

Steps

Close your eyes and sit in Padmasana and use the right thumb to close your right nostril. Inhale slowly through the left nostril, taking in as much air as you can to fill your lungs. Remove the thumb from right nostril and exhale. While exhaling, use the middle finger to close your left nostril and inhale with right nostril. Remove the thumb from the right nostril and exhale.

Reps Perform for 2–5 minutes

2. BHRAMARI

BHRAMARI pranayam

This pranayama obtain its name from the Bhramari, the black Indian bee. This resembles the typical humming sound of a bee!

What it does

Calms your mind down immediately and is one of the best breathing exercises to distress as it free the mind of anxiety, anger, or agitation.

Steps to practice Bhramari Pranayama:

Close your ears with thumbs and place index fingers on the temple.

Close eyes with the other three fingers. Carefully inhale through the nose and hold for a few seconds. Keep the mouth closed, exhale by making a humming sound.

Breathe in again and out and do the same pattern for around 6–7 times.

3. UJJAYI PRANAYAMA

Also known as ocean breath, this breathing technique involves a soft hissing sound during inhalation. UJJAYI PRANAYAMA

What it does

The sound vibrations of this pranayama improves the focus of mind can help cure thyroid and reduce snoring.

Steps

Begin by inhaling and exhaling naturally. Bend down head, blocking the free flow of air and inhale as long, making a sound from throat.

Hold for 2–5 seconds. Close right nostril with right thumb while exhaling and breathe out through the left nostril.

Reps 10–12 times in as much time you need

4. KAPALBHATHI

Known as the skull shining breathing technique, this strong deep breathing exercise is synonymous with Baba Ramdev for most of us.

What it does

This pranayama can enhance the functioning of all abdominal organs, reduces belly fat, lead to weight loss, and balances sugar levels in your body.

Steps are:

1. Sit in a comfortable yogic posture.

2. Make a suitable hand gesture.

3. Inhale deep (First breath).

4. Exhale active & Inhale passively.

5. Repeat 5–10 times & Relax'

5. BHASTRIKA

The forceful breathing exercise clears up your respiratory system and is characterized by sounds like a flame burning below a furnace.

What it does

Complete this breathing technique to strengthen your lungs, burn excess fat, improve physical and mental ability.

How to Perform Bhastrika

Sit in Padmasana (Lotus Pose).

Take a deep breath and fill lungs with air. Release the breath after counting till five.

Listen to the songs birds or instrumental slow music

Now begin the technique by inhaling and exhaling with force.

To begin with, perform at least 21 times (one round of inhalation and exhalation will count as one time).

Always check with your doctor before performing any breathing exercises. One may advise against doing if you suffer from any health issues.

Meditation Points to be noted while performing OMKAR pranayama

OM chanting should be rhythmic and slow while chanting one should not break the pitch. While inhaling take a deep breath, while exhaling try to open the mouth in O' shape slowly then pronounce M' and continue the chanting till it is possible as long one as one can breathe and while chanting OM out abdomen should contract inwards. The yoga sutras of Patanjali convey OM is the symbol of God.

Benefits of OMKAR Pranayama

1. This Pranayama we get ample blood supply to the brain.

2. This Pranayama purifies thoughts; it relaxes, rejuvenates the body and mind.

3. Studies have shown that this Pranayama reduces stress-related problems like hypertension, anxiety, and depression.

Anyone can practice OMKAR Pranayama.

CHAPTER 5

Workouts

Types of Workouts to Improve Health and Fitness Levels

Endurance Training also is known as aerobic exercise, helps develop stamina.

Strength Training also is known as resistance training, causes contractions of the muscles via external resistance.

Static Stretching are those in which you stand, sit or lie still and hold a single position or period that is 45 seconds.

Fitness Terms Everyone Should Know before They Step Foot in a Gym

We have decoded common fitness terms for you so that you can work out with confidence and get the most out of your fitness routine.

1. Active Recovery

This is one way to spend your "rest". We recommend light walking or gentle yoga. The reason why you might want to do this is do gentle movement into these days can help with circulation and reduce muscle fatigue.

2. Aerobic Exercise

During aerobic exercise, your body uses oxygen for energy, like a long walk, jogging, running, or bicycle ride.

3. Anaerobic Exercise

On the other hand, your anaerobic energy system is more stressful as these are short intervals of work used to improve speed, stamina, and power.

when you do high-intensity workouts that shoot up your heart rate.

4. Gym Camp

It often starts with running outside the Gym, followed by a wide variety of interval training, including bodyweight moves like push-ups and sit-ups, and various types of intense exercises.

5. Circuit

Think of this as the next round of exercises. For example, one circuit consists of 15 push-ups, 15 plank, and 20 jump squats. "You are working from one exercise to the other with rest in between each exercise.

6. Compound Exercises

A compound exercise is a move that incorporates multiple muscle groups, like deadlifts, chest, and biceps. It may also refer to two moves being together, like a bicep curl to a shoulder press. Compound exercise increases overall muscle mass and burning calories (because they require more effort to complete), as opposed to isolation exercises, which focus on working just one muscle group (like a bicep curl/triceps).

7. Cool-Down

This is what you do at the end of your workout is cool off the body and bring your body back to a resting state by lowering your heart rate.

8. Cross-Training

Cross-training means mixing in different workouts and training methods rather than just one type of workout. This will help to create a well-balanced fitness plan, but it can help you reach specific goals. For example, if you're getting ready to run a race or swim or walk, you will want to cross-train with strength, training methods, and yoga workouts, which will complement your running and help improve your performance and decrease injury by building muscle and increasing flexibility.

9. Soreness

The soreness you feel the day or two after a exercise. The muscle then repairs and rebuilds and that shows you get stronger muscles.

10. Warm-Up

This is what you should be doing before exercise to raise your heart rate and body temperature for the workout. During this type of warm-up, you should do stretches and light exercises without stopping. This helps increase mobility.

11. HIIT

HIIT stands for high-intensity interval training. This refers to quick, severe burst of exercise, followed by short recovery periods and this type of training keeps your heart rate up. This workout is great for burning fat.

12. Interval Training

An interval is a activity or a period of rest. While this often refers to HIIT workouts, you can implement intervals in pretty much any workout and maybe 30–40 seconds of work and 30–40 seconds of rest, or 15 minutes of work and 2 minutes of rest—it depends on what your goals are.

13. Isometrics

Isometric exercises a position under pressure and stay in that position for a set amount of time and they are a great way to build strength.

14. Reps

Shorthand for repetitions. Saying 10 repetitions means doing an exercise 10 times.

15. Resistance

Resistance means how much weight your muscles are working against to complete a workout. That can mean anywhere from your bodyweight to a set of five or ten pound dumbbells.

16. Sets

A set refers to number of times you repeat a given number of reps and for example, one set might be 15 reps of push-ups—repeating for three sets means you are repeating three times.

17. Steady-State Cardio

Steady-state cardio refers to exercise where you set pace at a adequate intensity, like a long run or swimming.

18. Strength Training

Strength training means using resistance to work your muscles; that can be your bodyweight, dumbbells, etc. The goal of this type of workout is to increase muscle mass and getting stronger helps improve everyday performance, and increase your metabolism.

19. Super Set

Super setting means pairing two exercises and doing back-to-back. There are a few ways to do these: You could save time by working two different muscle groups (like arms and shoulders) so you don't need to rest in between exercises because one muscle group is recovering while the other is working.. Another option is to pair "push" and "pull" movements—for example, a push – up and a pull-up.

A gymnasium, is derived from the ancient Greek gymnasium. They are commonly found in fitness centers, and as activity and learning activities in educational institutions. "Gym" is used for "fitness center", which is an area for indoor or outdoor activities. A gym is a place with several equipment and machines used by different people to do different exercises.

Inside a gymnasium are barbells, running paths are used as exercises. Today, gymnasium are common place in the India, and the rest of the world. They are in virtually all U.S. colleges and high schools, almost all middle schools and elementary schools. These facilities are used for physical education. The number of gyms in the U.S. has more than doubled since the late 1990s.

CHAPTER 6

You Can Be Your Trainer

"Success is neither magical nor mysterious.

Success is the natural consequence of consistently applying the fundamentals."

...Jim Rohn

Can I Be My Trainer/Physical Instructor?

With commitment, you can learn how to be your trainer. Becoming your trainer/physical instructor takes a few hours and the payment is huge. You'll gain all of the essential skills to get your mind, body in shape, and lose weight along the way.

Is it good to have a personal trainer in the gym? Why

Personal trainers will coach, push, and inspire you more. Working with a trainer allows you the freedom to create your workout schedule regarding your goals.

Important steps for a personal trainer

1. **Set a Goal.** During this first step, you define and write out your goals. This step is the most component of your plan to get fit, improve your sports performance like running or lose weight so grab a pen and paper and begin your journey.

2. **Improve Your Diet.** Weight loss can happen in the gym or home, but the biggest changes usually happen when you change your diet and all diets that work are based on the

same principle. You do need to make some adjustments for your calorie intake and get enough protein and carbohydrates for weight loss.

3. **Create Your Exercise Plan**. When you become your trainer/physical instructor, you will combine both aerobic workouts and strength training workouts to get lean and fit. Every workout should have the intensity and consistency of your sessions.

4. **Schedule Meals and Workouts**. The best professional coaches create an organized weekly program for their clients and this step is essential. Schedule one hour each week to set up your eating plan including meals, snacks and workout routines for the week. Post using print-outs/photos can make the job easier where you see it every day.

5. **Motivate Yourself to Stay on Track**. Just like any personal trainer, you'll experience moments of challenge and you will want to give up and you'll have to rely on yourself and your commitment to keeping yourself going. Personal trainers have particular methods they use to keep their clients on track. **(Fig 16)**

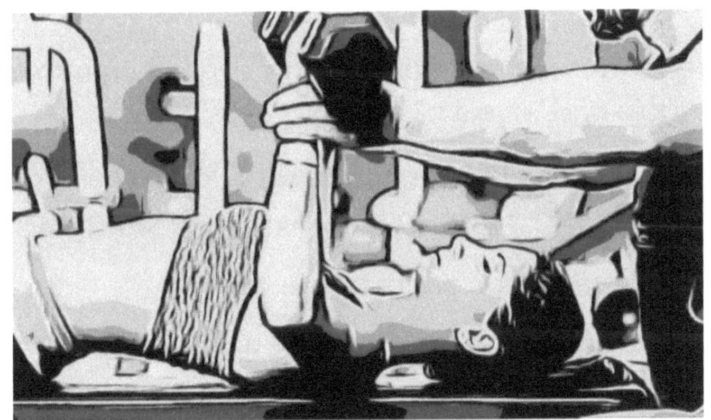

6. **Set Specific, Targeted, Achievable, Motivating Goals**. Ask yourself the following what do I want to achieve with my fitness. Be able to run a marathon in under one-two hours.

Lose weight? Feel better? Walk longer? Run 5 kilometers? Once you have that goal in place, you need to figure out if it is achievable. Can you look like a model? Possible? Then fine. Will you be able to run 5 miles in less than two hours? Maybe not. Or it might take several years to get to that point. Make sure your goals are within the time you've allotted.

7. **Evaluate Every Week**. Goals should be measurable, if you're on the road to success. For example, weighing yourself once a week tells you at a glance if you're heading in the right direction and write it down.

8. **Take Measurements**. It's really important to look at measurements and most good personal trainers will take body measurements during your first session.

Abdominal: Waist: _ Shoulder: _ Hip:

Chest: _

Thigh (Mid):

Arm:(L) (R): _

Blood Pressure:

Make sure to take these measurements every month to track your progress again and write it all down.

1. **Fill Out an Initial Fitness Assessment.** When you're developing your fitness program, ask yourself a few key questions

    A. Where do you prefer to exercise

        i. Outside – Some people prefer jogging/running half an hour prior to gym which helps to reduce the weight.

        ii. Inside

        iii. Combination

   B. What time do you like to exercise?

       i. Early Morning

      ii. Morning

     iii. Midmorning

     iv. Late Afternoon

      v. Evening

     vi. Late Evening

   C. How many times per week can you exercise?

      More than a two hours is more than enough for light weight training

   D. How much time can you spend daily on exercise/ training?

      Make it routine to exercise daily.

   E. What are the best days for you to exercise?

      Monday, Wednesday, Friday Or Tuesday, Thursday, Saturday, that is every alternate day so that body gets enough time for rest.

2. **Learn to do Your Routine Correctly.** Plan your specific exercises and learn how to do them correctly. There are many websites and Youtube that have helpful instructional videos on how to do exercises correctly.

3. **Plan next exercise as You Rest.**Instead of counting seconds between sets, use the time to start planning your next move and grab the weights you'll be using next; check how many repetitions you did during your last workout.

If you paid for the gym

1. **Put Pressure On Yourself**. Money can be motivating factor so you're less inclined to skip a session for which you've already paid.

2. **Keep Off Distractions at the Gym and stay awake always.** Having a trainer is the best way to keep people from interrupting your routine, because people are less likely to chat with you when you're busy and that way you can always listen to music during your workout.

3. **Buy Key Fitness Equipment from Online/Offline.** You can get a treadmill, bike or any workout gear by looking online. Do your research to find good quality units, and make sure to test one first then buy.

CHAPTER 7

Abdomen Workouts

"To succeed in your mission, you must have single-minded devotion to your goal."

...Dr. APJ Abdul Kalam

How to Do the Best Abs Workout Circuits for Upper Abs, Lower Abs to Sculpt a Rock-Hard Six-Pack

If you're looking to train your abs, there is a variety of exercises that will help you achieve that goal and the location of your abs means that they are worked hard to hit both the upper and lower body.

Your goal is a six-pack or just a more definition around your midsection, compound lifts like squats, overhead presses and deadlifts will help get you there, and they'll build strength to achieve a model-like six-pack.

The really good news is that you don't need access to a gym to complete these workouts, you can keep pursuing your six-pack dream you can get into shape at home during lockdown with minimal equipment.

How To Do Each Abs Workout. These are the 24 exercises for abdomen workout

Upper Abs Workout 1

1. Dumbbell crunch (Fig 17)

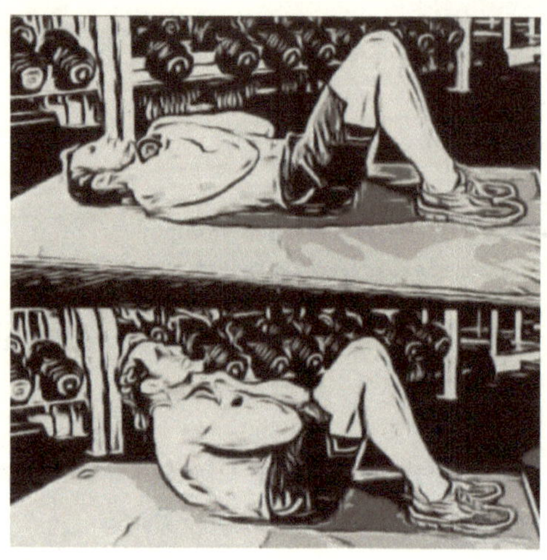

Reps 10 **Rest** 20sec

Lie on your back, holding a dumbbell or weight plate across your chest in both hands and raise your torso, then lower it, maintaining tension in your uppers abs throughout.

2. Modified V-sit (Fig 18)

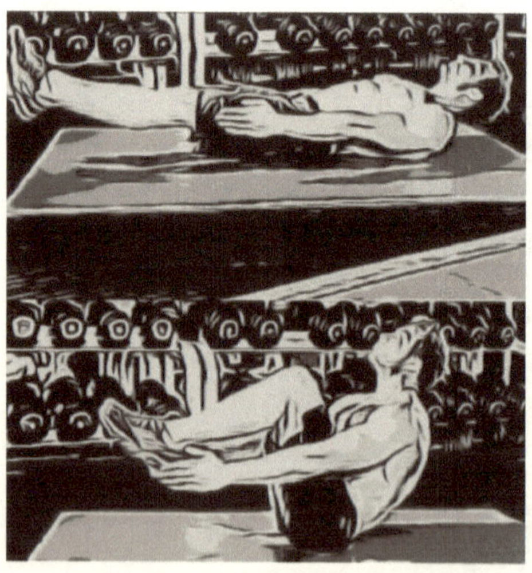

Reps 12 **Rest** 10sec

Lie with your legs raised off the floor and extended away from you so they're parallel with the floor, and your arms straight by your sides, held off the floor. Keep your arms straight as you raise your torso and bring your legs in, bending at the knees, so that your chest meets your knees at the top.

3. Crunch (Fig 19)

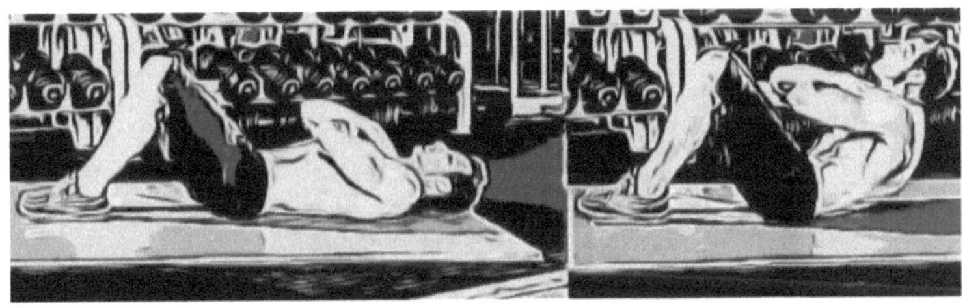

Reps 20 **Rest** 90sec

Lie on your back with your knees bent and feet planted, and your arms crossed across your chest. Raise your torso using your abs, then lower. Your upper abs will already be close to fatigue but try to hold the top position of each rep for at least one/two second to make them work as hard as possible.

Lower Abs Workout

4. Hanging leg raise(Fig 20)

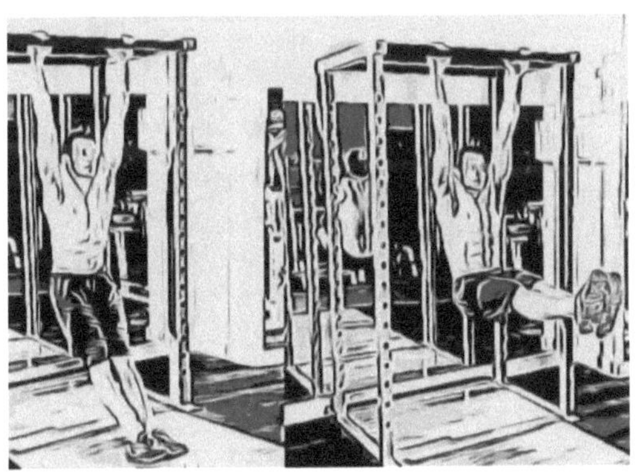

Reps 10 **Rest** 20sec

This tough exercise sets the tone for what is going to be a brutal workout involving different hanging exercises. Start in a dead hang with your legs straight and your knees and ankles touching. Keep them together as your use your lower abs to raise them, then lower back to the start under control.

5. Hanging knee raise twist (Fig 21)

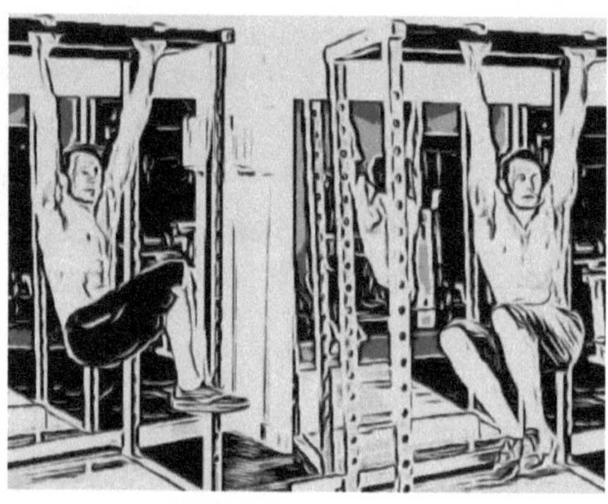

Reps 10 each side **Rest** 10sec

Start in a dead hang with your legs straight and knees together. Twist your body and raise your knees to one side, then return to the start, continue and then alternating sides.

6. Hanging knee raise (Fig 22)

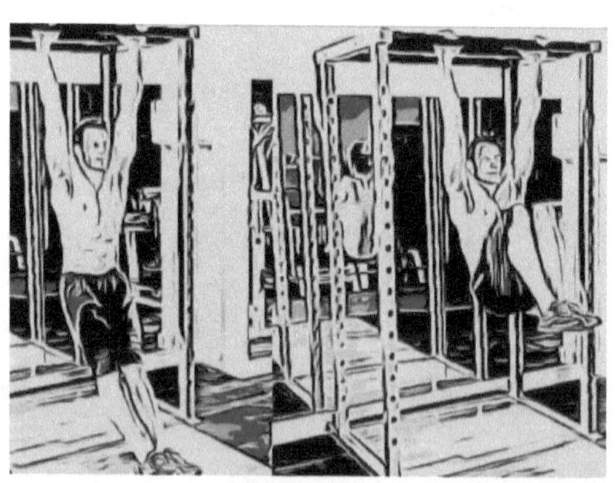

Reps 15 **Rest** 10sec

This slightly easier variation on the hanging leg raise still puts a lot of pressure on your lower abs. Start in a dead hang and raise your knees powerfully to activate more of the muscle fibres in the lower abs. Lower back to the start under control to prevent swinging.

7. Garhammer raise (Fig 23)

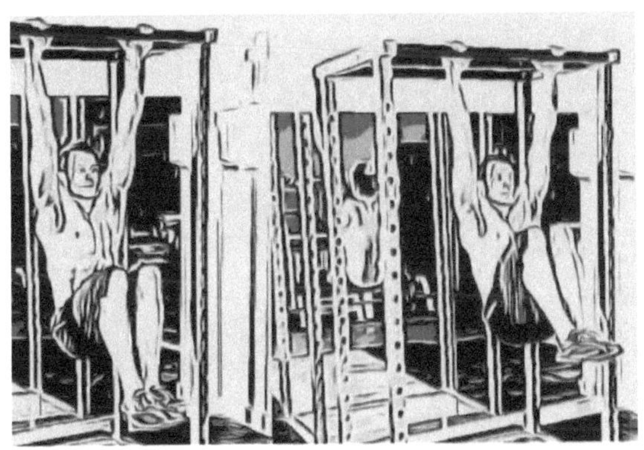

Reps 20 **Rest** 90sec

Start hanging from the bar but with your knees already raised to around your midsection, then lift them as high as you can and lower back to the start under control.

8. Decline plank with foot touch (Fig 24)

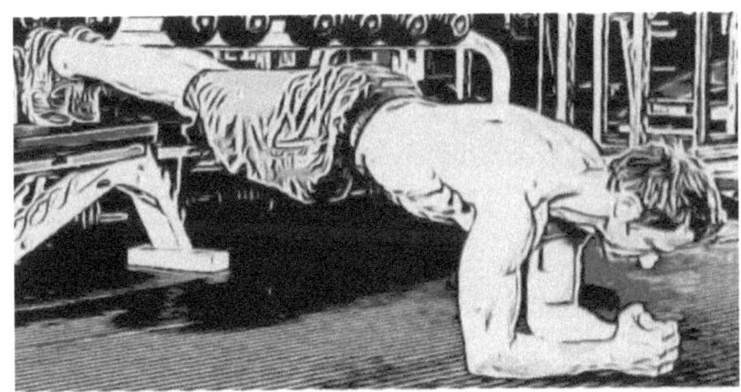

Reps 10 each side **Rest** 10sec

Get into a decline plank position, supporting yourself on your forearms with your feet raised on a bench. Your body should form a straight line from heels to head and the aim is to maintain that position throughout the exercise. Lift one foot off the bench and move it to the side to touch the floor, then return it to the bench. Continue, alternating sides.

9. Seated Russian twist (Fig 25)

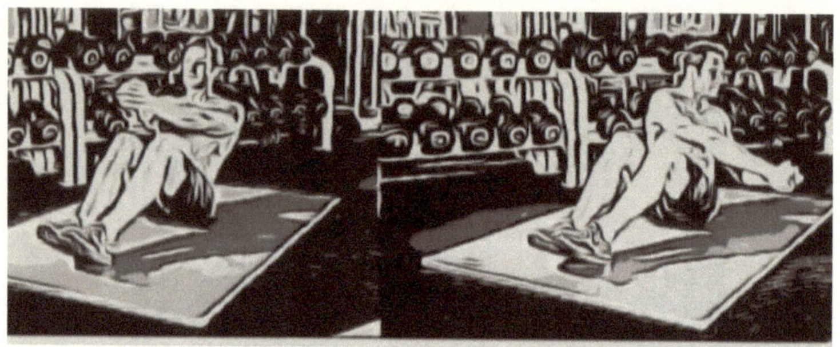

Reps 12 each side **Rest** 10sec

Sit on the floor with your knees bent and heels on the ground. Your torso should be at the top of the crunch position, forming a 45° angle to the ground and twist your torso from side to side, moving in a smooth and controlled manner.

10. Bicycle crunches (Fig 26)

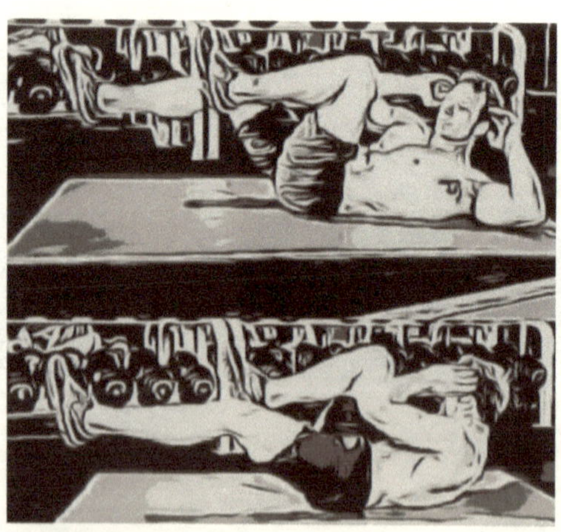

Reps 15 each side **Rest** 10–20sec

Lie on your back with your hands by your temples and your legs raised with your knees bent at a 90° angle. Bring your right knee up towards your chest while raising torso and twisting so your left elbow comes to meet your knee. Then lower and do the same on the opposite side. Keep your shoulders and feet off the ground to force your abs to work hard

11. Plank (Fig 27)

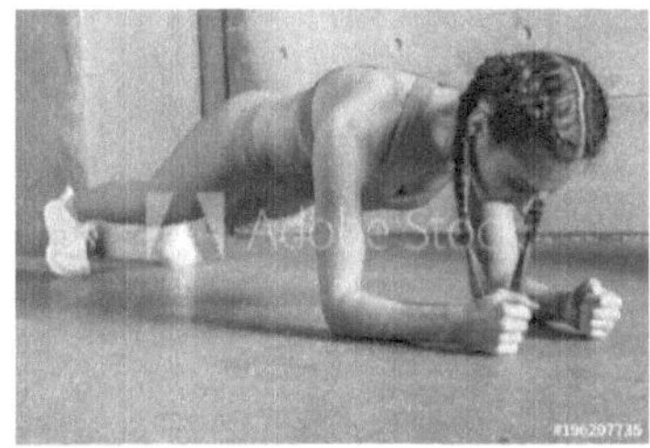

Get into pushup position and bend your elbows to lower your forearms to the floor. Hold the position with abs braced.

Abs Training Tips

The abs should be trained every day. Two or four abs workouts a week might be optimal for most people and breaking it up into separate days is one good option.

12. Abdomen Wheel Rollout (Fig 28)

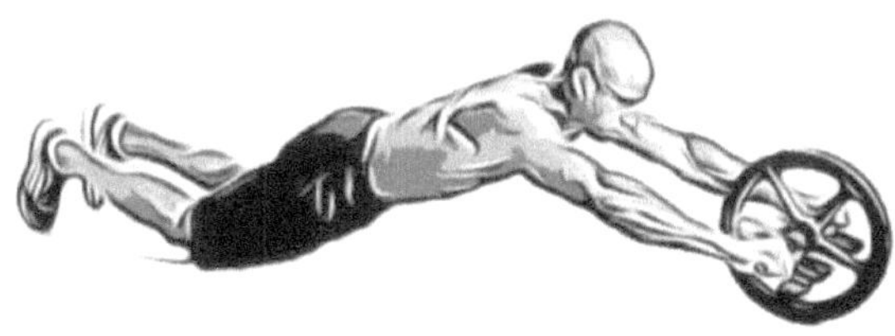

Kneel on the floor and hold an abdomen wheel beneath your shoulders. Brace your abs and roll the wheel forward until you feel

you're about to lose tension in your core and your hips. Roll yourself back to start. Do as many reps as you can.

13. Arms-High Partial Situp (Fig 29)

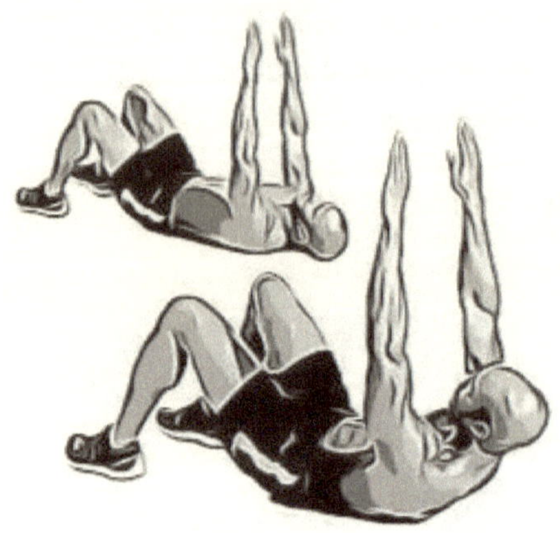

Lie on your back, knees bent at 90 degrees, and raise your arms straight overhead, keeping them pointing up throughout the exercise. Sit up halfway, then steadily return to the floor. That's one rep then repeat the exercise again.

14. Barbell Rollout (Fig 30)

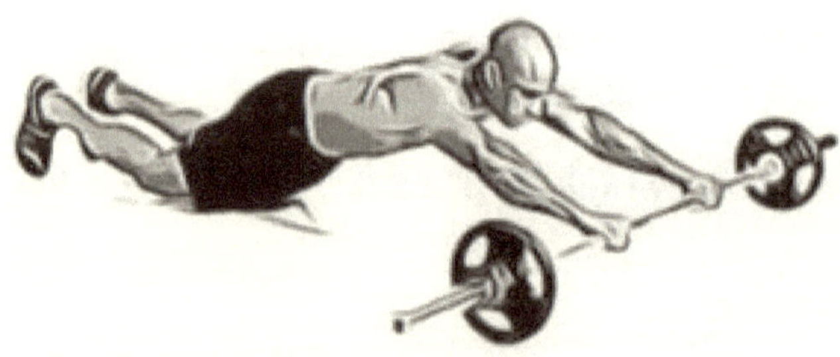

Load the barbell with 10-pound plates and kneel on the floor behind it. Your shoulders should be over the bar move your abs and roll the bar forward, reaching in front of you until you feel your hips and roll yourself back.

15. Barbell Russian Twist (Fig 31)

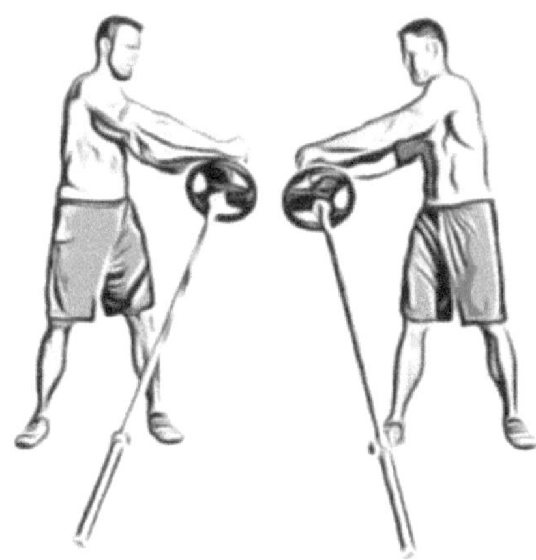

Grasp the barbell near the very end again—this time with both hands. Stand with 1 feet at width and swing the bar to your left, then swing to your right.

16. Leg Raise Combo (Fig 32)

Suspend yourself over the parallel bars at a dip. Bend your knees slightly and raise your legs in front of you until they're parallel to the floor and this will build you a 6 pack.

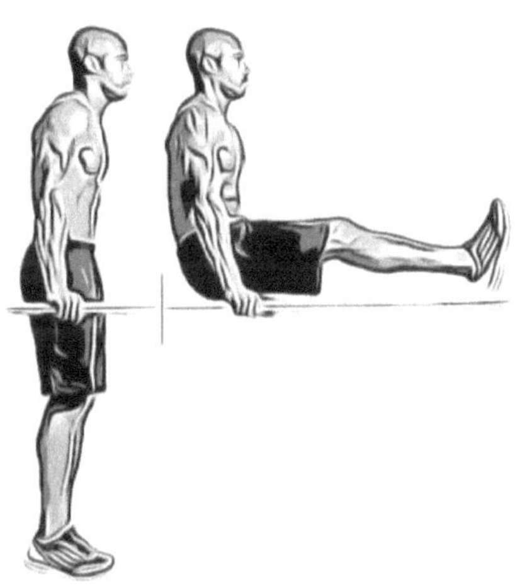

17. Kick like scissor (Fig 33)

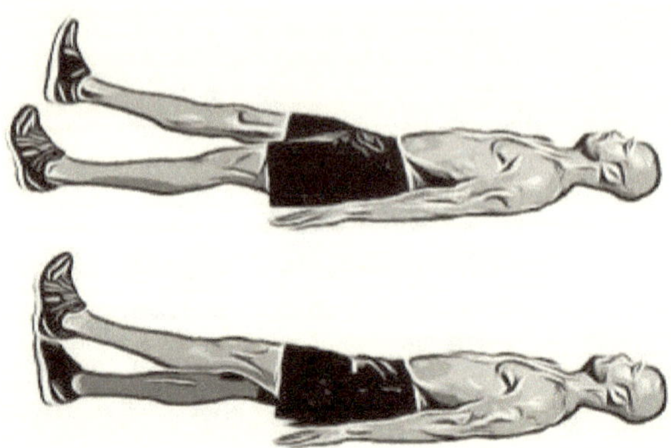

Lie on your back with legs straight and arms extend out at your sides. Lift your heels about 6–8 inches off the floor and rapidly kick your feet up and down in a quick in scissor-like motion.

18. Front Squat (Fig 34)

Set a barbell on a rack at about shoulder height and grasp the bar with hands at shoulder width and raise your elbows until your upper arms are parallel to the floor. Take the bar out of the rack and let it rest on your finger tips—as long as your elbows stay up, you'll be able to balance the bar. Step back and set your feet at shoulder width with toes turned out slightly. Squat as low as you can until you feel the weight.

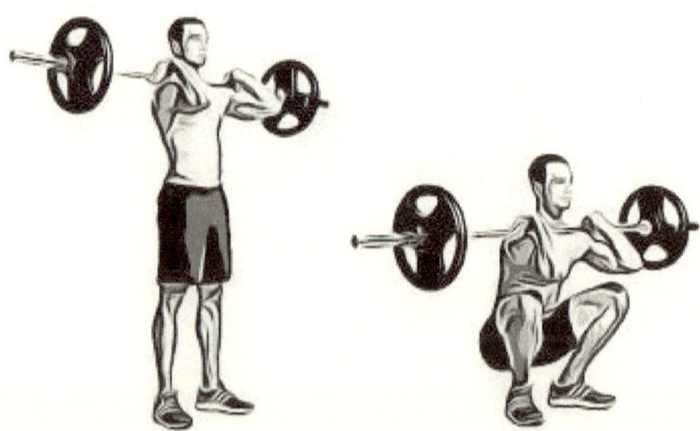

19. Leg Raise (Fig 35)

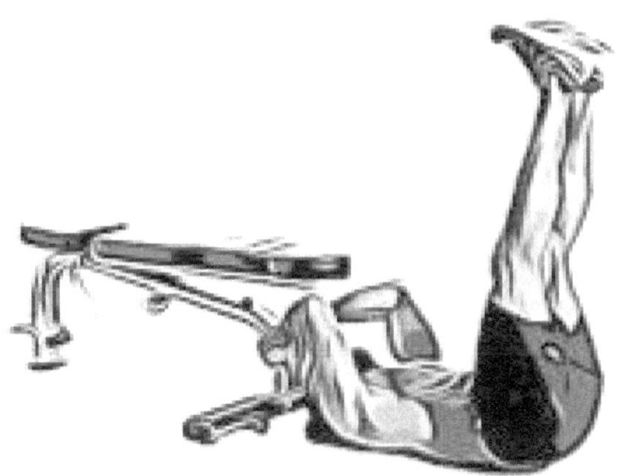

Lie on the floor and hold onto a bench or the legs of a heavy chair for support and keeping your legs straight and raise them up until they're 90^0 to the floor. Lower back down, but stop just short of the floor to keep tension on your abs.

20. Pull-up to Knee Raise (Fig 36)

Hang from a pull-up bar with hands outside shoulder width and palms facing away from you. Pull yourself up until your chin is over the bar and then raise your knees to your chest.

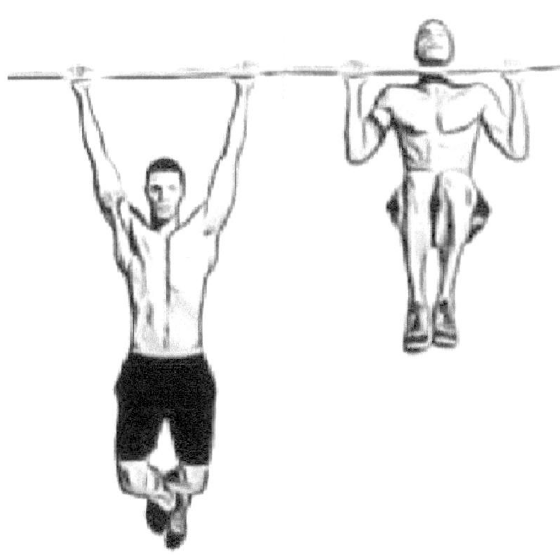

21. Side Plank (Fig 37)

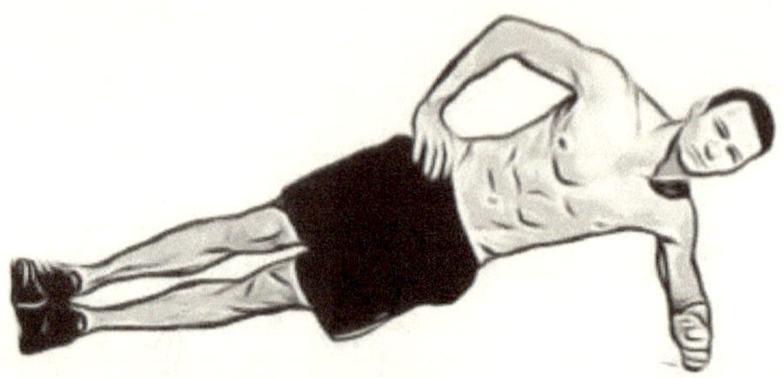

Lie on your left side resting your left forearm on the floor for support. Raise your hips up so your body forms a straight line and your abs— your weight should be on your left forearm and the edge of your left foot. Hold the position with abs in position.

22. Sit up and move forward (Fig 38)

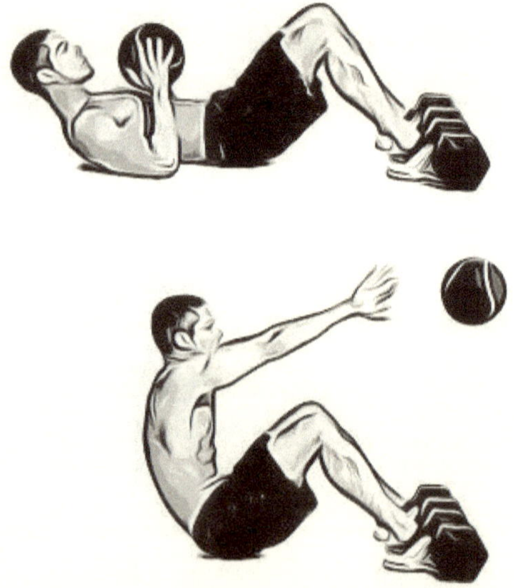

Hold your feet under something sturdy/hard for support, and lie back on the floor a few feet away from a wall. Sit up and push the ball against wall.

23. Weighted Sit up (Fig 39)

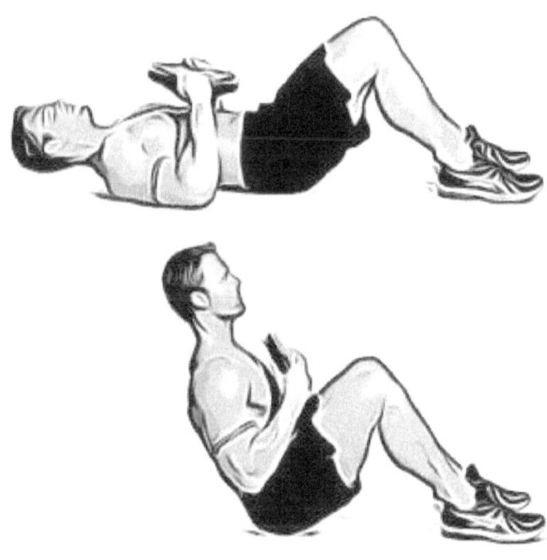

Lie on the floor holding a weight plate at your chest. Bend your knees 90 degrees with feet on the floor and tuck your chin to your chest and sit up all the way.

Please Note: Stop this exercise if your feeling discomfort or please contact your Doctor.

Running

"I love to strengthen myself with a healthy diet, plenty of exercises and maintaining a strong connection to myself."

...Renae A.Sauter

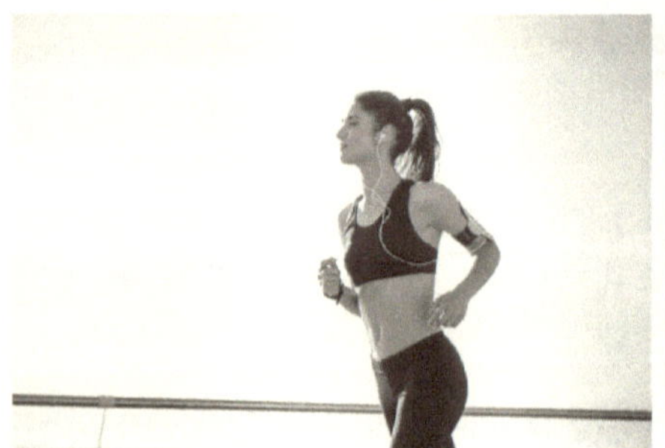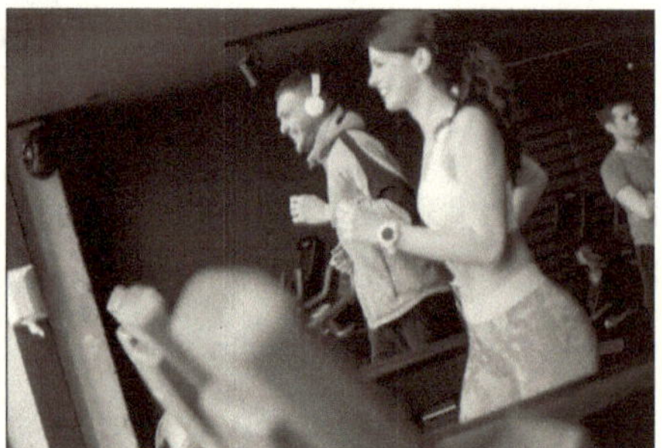

Benefits of Running

Running **(Fig 40)** is actually a great way to increase your overall level of health. Research shows that running can raise your levels of good cholesterol while also helping you increase lung function and use. In addition, running can also boost your immune system and lower your risk of developing blood clots. During lockdown everybody prefers indoor activity like running on treadmill machine **(Fig 41)**.

Running

Within 30 minutes:

You don't have to wait for months to see the benefits and your daily dose of running will start showing the benefits instantaneously.

1. Studies has shown that exercise can instantly boost mood and help you start your day in full force. Running is probably the best way and 20 minutes of running can work to lift your mood. Here's another study that found exercise can be as good as antidepressant.

2. Running prepares you to cope with daily stress and challenges.

3. Running also helps with anxiety disorder and panic attacks. They found that more physically active people were less likely to panic in fearful situations.

4. It will regulate your blood pressure.

5. 30 minutes of running combined with the warm ups and stretching (45 minutes in total) will boost your metabolism for the next 12 hours.

After 24 hours:

6. A study found out that employees are happier and more efficient at workplace on days when they exercise. The study talks about the workplace but we can safely assume that the better mood and performance will help in all areas of life.

7. Running will make you think highly of yourself and studies found that exercise boosts people's confidence and improve their body image.

8. A study suggests that running or exercise can increase self-esteem in children or young people. High energy level improve our confidence.

9. You will learn information faster at office, in classroom, or any other environment. A study looked at different recreational activities and their impact after a learning period and the group that was made to run performed better than any other group in the study.

10. Running results in increased cortisol levels that is needed for better memory.

11. Running helps you burn a lot of calories.

12. Running has greatly improved your sleeping habits on your mind and body are getting the much-needed rest. A relaxed mind is a powerful mind and it results in better psychological function. Running will help you sleep more easily.

After a month

13. We just discussed some benefits but the one will start when you have made it a routine.

14. Running keep you more focused and awake. You will adapt to changes and deal with new challenges.

15. You are inspiring others to exercise and you have become an inspiration for your friends and family members. Sharing your daily routine and milestones will push your friends to start running. Studies have shown that an extra kilometer/miles by a friend can inspire others to improve upon the distance of kms/miles or time and this is especially true for men. Besides, the positive changes in your mood and encourage your friends to follow your footstep and run more.

16. Running can help you curb the bad habits or addictions like smoking, or excessive drinking and you might even start to like vegetables and fruits. It's not just the diet but you will start to make healthier choices in other aspects of life.

17. Running will boost your energy levels and that tiredness. In a study, the group that exercised felt "much better" compared to those who did not exercise. A 6 week trial of young adults who reported feeling of tiredness found improvements in energy levels and a drop in fatigue.

18.   Mental illnesses and psychological disorders are less affected because of your running routine.

After 6 Months. Miles/kms are coming along nicely and running is not as hard as it used to be before.

19.   Running just 7 – 14 miles a week can keep your cholesterol levels in check.

20.   Training for your first marathon: This study confirms that it can trim up to 4 years off the arterial age that is, your arteries will be 4 years younger after a few months of long distance running.

21.   Running will gradually affect and improve your diet and lifestyle habits. You will manage to cut down your booze intake and a study found that the exercise group managed to make healthy changes to their drinking habits..

1 year: It is almost a year since you started running that's quite an achievement and the rewards are you are stronger and healthier.

22.   Strong knees or back can mean so much especially as you age and your knees will actually get healthier because of your regular running routines.

23.   Running will also strengthen your thighs, quads, or hamstrings which are some of the most important muscles in your body.

24.   The benefits will multiply if you are combining aerobic with meditation has it will considerably reduce depression .

After one decade of running.

25.   Luckily, your legs, knees, and backs are stronger and you can considerably improve your bone health through running.

26. Running strengthens muscles that are responsible for supporting your stomach and spine and it makes it easy to maintain a healthy, upright posture.

27. Your heart is more healthier because running or aerobics are considered the best form of exercise for cardiovascular health.

28. Running is also helping you deal with emotional pain or suffering from the past. A study found that marathon runners tend to forget physical pain after six months..

After 25 years it has been a long time. Keeping up with your running routine as only 20% adults in US meet the physical activity recommendation.

29. You look much younger than your age and this is because of regular physical activity that slows down biological aging and studies suggests that high levels of physical activity can reduce up to 9 year of biological aging.

30. Skin is usually the first thing that give away your age. A study found that 40 years old people who regularly exercise had skin like 20 or 30 years old.

You will live longer as scientists followed 1000 adults for 21 years. All these adults were aged 50 or older. After 21 years 85% runners were alive while just 66% non-runners managed to survive. We have discussed how running can help you adapt healthy eating habits, quit smoking, improve your sleep, and mental health and all these changes will definitely contribute to longevity.

Living your life to the fullest/above 60/70/80 years:

31. It will improve the quality of life. For example, you have 41% lower risk of getting cataracts, which is the leading cause of vision loss and blindness in elderly. Moderate (walking) and vigorous (running) exercise were both significantly associated with lower cataract risk and their effects similar.

32. A study of 70 years old participants who have a lifelong habit of doing exercise found that their heart, lungs, and muscles are as good as those of 40 years old.

33. Dementia or brain diseases are a common problem in the older age and, you are far less likely to suffer from this problem even in your 80s.It means you will have a better working memory in the old age.

CHAPTER 9

Walking

"Walking is man's best medicine."

...Hippocrates

How Walking Can Help You Lose Weight and Abdomen Fat (Fig 42)

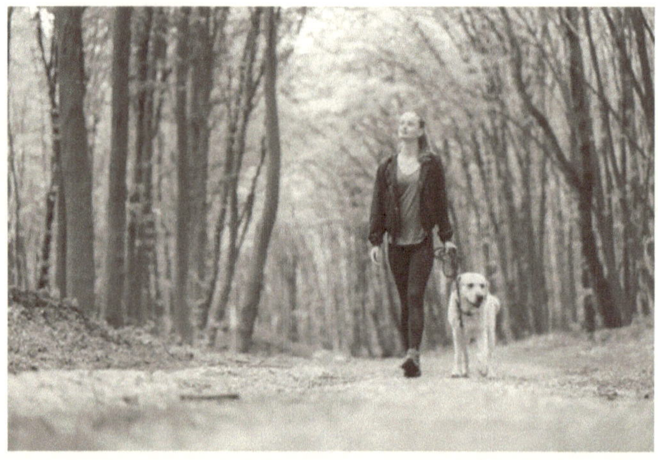

If you want to stay fit and healthy, it's important to exercise regularly and it is beneficial for weight loss and maintenance. Walking is a great form of physical activity that's free, low risk and accessible to most people.

Walking Burns Calories. Your body needs energy (in the form of calories) to move, breathe, think and function normally. Daily calorie needs vary from person to person and are affected by things like your weight, sex, genes and activity level and it's well known that you need to burn more calories than you consume to lose weight .

It Helps To Maintain Lean Muscle. When people cut calories and lose weight, they often lose muscle in addition to body fat and this helps you burn more calories each day.

It can reduce age-related muscle loss, helping you retain more of your muscle strength and function.

Study suggests that walking can be recommended to women with obesity. Walking exercise is effective in to maintain proper weight.

Brisk walking: Brisk walking is defined as walking continuously for at least 10 minutes in the past 4 weeks.

Benefits of walking

1. Heart health is huge in enjoying a healthier lifestyle.

2. It prevents major diseases.

3. Walking reduces the risk of blood pressure and stroke.

4. It reduces cholesterol.

5. The pain in the joints and bones is reduced.

6. Weight is kept in control with daily walking.

Walkers have fewer incidences of diabetes and other diseases. They live longer and get mental and spiritual health benefits.

Morning walks keeps us energetic whole day due to the abundance oxygen. This supplies good amount of oxygen to the internal organs and morning walk is a good weight loss tip; this will help us to keep body fit and healthy.

An evening walk is a activity that can help us clear away all the negative/stressful thoughts that may come across the course of the day. Taking a walk half an hour after we've eaten can help us sleep well because one feels the relaxed state of mind after the evening walk.

Important points

- Walk Away from arguments that leads you to nowhere.

- Walk Away from people who deliberately put you down.

- Walk Away from failures and fears that hold back your dreams.

- Walk Away from people who do not care and are opportunistic.

- The more you Walk Away from things that poison your soul, the happier your life will be. Give Yourself a Walk towards love, peace, kindness and goodness

CHAPTER 10

Dance

"Blessed are the people who are living dreams they didn't know they had. Dreams they never dreamed. Dreams that came to life because they followed their intuition."

...Renae. A. Sauter

Dance for Health: Improving Fitness (Fig 43)

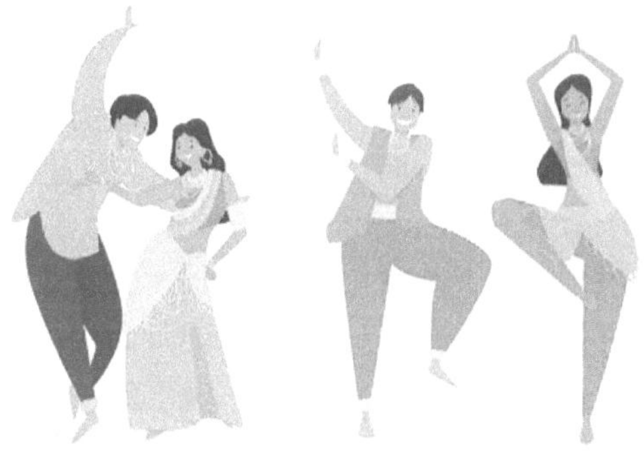

1. Bollywood dance.

In recent years, Bollywood dance classes have been offered in many areas of the world. Bollywood dance is a form of exercise, appealing to those interested in fitness and in losing weight. The program will help you increase your health and fitness levels, develop flexibility and grace, increase stamina and endurance levels, and strengthen your heart. This program will help you lose weight and increase your metabolism, helping you burn off extra calories all this while having entertainment. Bollywood Music and dance is a very strong part of our movies and they're part of our storytelling. We come across songs which emotions, devotion, love, agony, pain, separation. (Aishwarya Rai, 22 October 2003). However, dancing is an exercise if it is done regularly, not occasionally.

2. Zumba (Fig 44)

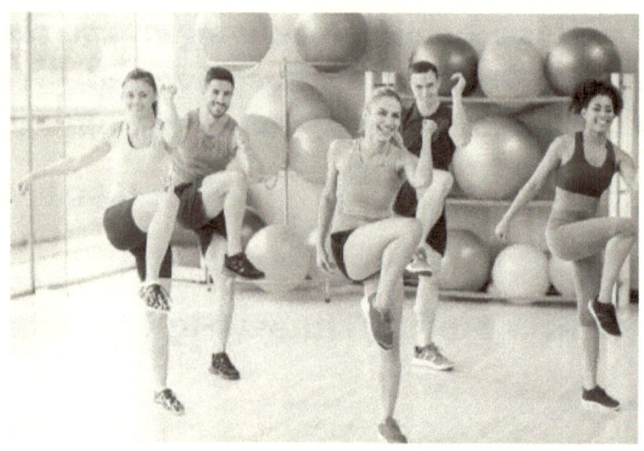

Zumba is a feel-good way to improve your fitness and an effective way of exercise into your daily routine. Zumba is all about burning calories, it has been found to help relieve stress, increase energy, and improve strength. It incorporates vigorous exercise and high-intensity movement which helps the body in getting shape and weight reduction. In between squats, twists, and multiple dance routines.

CHAPTER 11

Cycling

"Life is like riding a bicycle,

To keep your balance,

You must keep moving".

...Albert Einstein

Why Cycling

Health benefits of regular cycling

1. Increased cardiovascular fitness.

2. Increased muscle strength and flexibility.

3. Improved joint mobility.

4. Bicycling has been proven to boost your brain health, blood flow, memory, and overall function

5. Improved posture and coordination.

6. Strengthened bones.

7. Decreased body fat levels.

8. Cycling helps your lung capacity and lung function improve.

9. Cycling helps riders feel more relaxed throughout the day by relieving stress.

10. If you burn more calories than you consume, you will lose weight. When you are cycling for weight loss you should know that the more strenuous the cycling is, the more you'll burn the calories.

11. No noise and air pollution

CHAPTER 12

Swimming

"Physical fitness is the first requisite of happiness."

...Joseph Pilates

Why Do You Need to Swim? (Fig 45)

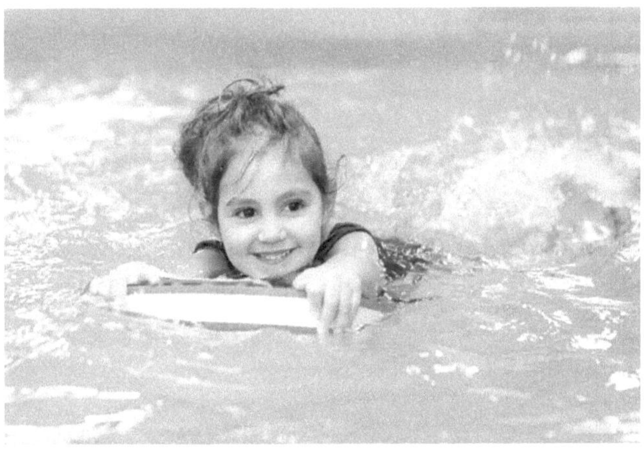

Swimming workouts burn fat, help you get stronger, fitter, and healthier. Swimming engages all of the major muscle groups, from your abdominals and back muscles to your arms, legs, and hips. It can compliment other exercises like walking and running as well.

1. A whole-body workout

Swimming engages every major muscle group, requiring a person to use their arms, legs, and stomach. Swimming also increases the heart rate without putting stress on the body, improves strength, enhances fitness, helps to manage/reduce weight.

2. Building cardiovascular strength

Cardiovascular exercise, involves the heart, lungs, and circulatory system and a thorough workout routine.

3. Suitable for all ages and fitness levels

Swimming allows a person to go at their own pace, and a person can learn to swim at a very young age, and most swimming pools have an area for beginners and people who prefer to swim slowly.

4. A great skill to have

The benefits of learning to swim safely and beyond mental and physical fitness and it may even be lifesaving.

5. Burning calories

Swimming is an excellent way to burn calories that is the amount burned depends on a person's weight and how vigorously they swim.

6. Helping to improve sleep

A study involving older adults with insomnia reported improved sleep in those who exercised regularly. Swimming may benefit those who seek better sleep.

7. Boosting moods

Swimming improve mood, and boost confidence and social skills, which can impact a person's self-esteem. People with dementia showed that those who swam regularly in 12 weeks showed an improvement in mood.

8. Managing stress

Exercise is a great way to relieve stress and anxiety and even 20 minutes of physical activity a week may help a person to feel more relaxed.

9. Great for kids

Kids need a minimum of 50–60 minutes of aerobics/swimming exercise each day.

CHAPTER 13

Weight Loss Tips

"You cannot change your future, but you can change your habits, and surely your habits will change your future." ...

...Dr. APJ Abdul Kalam

Weight loss tips: The weight loss industry is full of myths. In recent times, scientists have found several strategies that seem to be effective.

Here are weight loss tips that are evidence-based

1. Drink Water, Especially Before Meals

It is often claimed that drinking water can help with weight loss. Drinking water can boost metabolism over a period of 1–1.5 hours, helping you burn off a few more calories.

2. Eat Eggs For Breakfast

Eating whole eggs can have benefits, including helping you lose weight.

3. Drink Coffee (Preferably Black)

Coffee is loaded with antioxidants and can have numerous health benefits and studies show that the caffeine in coffee can boost metabolism and increase fat burning by up to 10–29%. Just make sure not to add sugar to your coffee.

4. Soups

Most foods with a low energy density that contain lots of water, such as vegetables and fruits. But you can also just add water to your food, making a soup.Some studies have shown that eating the same food turned into a soup rather than as solid food, makes people feel more satisfied and eat significantly fewer calories. Don't add too much fat to your soup, such as cream or coconut milk. Soups can be a weight loss diet.

Lemon Ginger diet soup

All you need to do is heat some chopped ginger, garlic, green chilies and onions in olive oil and add vegetable stock, once the onions are golden brown. Let the stock simmer for some time. Add lemon juice and salt to taste. Turn off the heat, once the stock has reduced to almost half and your diet soup is ready! It makes for the perfectly nutritious and healthy dinner recipe,

5. Chia Seeds

Chia seeds are the most nutritious foods on the planet.

This makes chia seeds a low-carb-friendly food. Due of its high fiber content, chia seeds can absorb up to 11–12 times their weight in water, and expanding in your stomach. Due to nutrient composition, chia seeds could be a useful part of your weight loss diet. Chia seeds are very high in fiber, which fills you up and reduces appetite and for therefore they can be useful in weight loss diet.

6. Drink Green Tea

Green tea also has benefits, like weight loss. Green tea is best superfoods contains powerful antioxidants called catechins, which are believed to work synergistically with caffeine to enhance fat burning. Recent studies show that green tea (either as a beverage or a green tea extract supplement) can help in weight loss. Combined with ginger and lemon, the tea prevents fat from accumulating in the body, fights cholesterol and improves immunity.

7. Ginger, lemon and honey

Drink warm water to the mixture of lemon, honey and ginger in empty stomach in the morning then you've got yourself a winning concoction, that can aid weight loss.

8. Try Intermittent Fasting

The procedure which makes the body light is fasting. Fasting is indicated in person with obesity etc. Intermittent fasting in which people cycle between periods of fasting and eating. Short-term studies suggest intermittent fasting is as effective for weight loss.

Almost everyone fast, some for health benefits, some for spiritual reasons, and some for religion.

a) Fasting allows one to control the appetite, which eventually helps to control the habit of overeating. This disciplines the mind to abstain from food.

b) Spiritually when one fasts, they refrain from all sorts of harmful eatables and fermented beverages that contain energies that change the balance of the body. This is a reminder that the person who lasts consciously and devotionally abstains from selfish and bodily desires, which is a act of controlled and inner development.

c) In medical terms the mechanics of the body related to digestion and excretion of food that is the digestive and excretory system is slowed down in its action allowing it to cleanse thoroughly, thereby improving circulation, stamina, and strength.

d) One can improve their self-confidence, get rid of the feeling of stress and tension by maintaining the food free days. Life begins to be full of positivity and this pure energy begins to spill throughout life.

e)   The best way to seek the maximum gains of fasting both spiritual and physical is when you know how and when it should be performed and with a thorough understanding of the mechanism.

The bottom line is **Don't Diet — Eat Healthily**. One of the worst side effects of dieting it causes muscle loss and metabolic slowdown. Focus should be on nourishing your body instead of starving it.

9. Cut Back on Sugar

Added sugar is one of the worst ingredients in the modern diet and most people consume way too much and studies show that sugar consumption is strongly associated with an increased risk of obesity, including type 2 diabetes and heart disease.

Avoid Sugary Drinks. Sugar is bad, but sugar in liquid form that is a soft drink is bad for health. Recent studies shows liquid sugar may be the single fattening factor and study showed that sugar-sweetened beverages are linked to a 60% increased risk of obesity in children.

10. Eat Less Refined Carbohydrates

Refined carbohydrates include sugar and grains that have been stripped of their fibrous, nutritious parts including white bread and pasta. Eating refined carbohydrates is strongly linked to obesity.

11. Use Smaller Plates

People using smaller plates has been shown eat fewer calories.

12. Simply eating less or calories can be very useful. Some studies show that taking pictures of your meals can help you lose weight.

13. Keep Healthy Food if you are Hungry

Keeping healthy food nearby can help prevent you from eating something unhealthy if you become excessively hungry like whole fruits, nuts, carrots, yogurt, and eggs.

14. Eat More Vegetables

Vegetables have several properties that make them effective for weight loss as they contain few calories and a lot of fiber. Their high water content gives them low energy, making them very filling. An example is eating vegetable salad with the meal. Vegetable juice like carrot juice.

a) Carrot Juice

Carrots juice is great for weight loss. A large glass of carrot juice will help you full until lunch. It is recommended that the best way to have carrots is in its raw form. Carrot juice is also known to increase bile secretion which helps in burning fat.

b) Cucumber Juice

Foods that have high water content are low in calories and due to its high water and fibre content, cucumber juice fills you up easily and so, it can be great meal filler. To cucumber juice, add some lime juice and few mint leaves to make a refreshing summer drink.

c) Amla Juice

Start your day with a glass of amla juice as it helps in keeping your digestive system on track throughout the day and accelerates metabolism, and this helps in burning fat quickly. To decrease weight it is often suggested to drink amla juice on an empty stomach. Add a drop of honey to amla that will keep you active and energetic throughout the day.

d) Gourd for Weight loss

Many people eat gourd daily as a medicine to cure their illnesses. It has vitamins, minerals, antioxidants, and fiber. It is excellent for digestive system and also reduces bad cholesterol. By adding gourd to your food, you can lose weight quickly. Gourd juice is useful in reducing weight. Gourd juice promotes a diuretic effect in the body, which helps in removing fat from the body.

e) Tulsi leaves

Tulsi helps in digestion and removes toxins out of your body, it regulates the metabolism of your body, helps in weight loss. It can be used as flavoring agent with green tea.

15. Drink Fruit Juices

a) **Pomegranate Juice:** Pomegranate juice is good for your skin and may also help in weight loss. Pomegranate juice also helps in suppressing your appetite, rich in anti-oxidants.

b) **Watermelon:** Watermelon juice is healthier.

c) **Orange juice:** Freshly squeezed orange juice could be healthier.

d) **Pineapple juice:** Pineapple juice helps in reducing belly fat.

16. Dry Fruits

Almonds, raisins, peanuts, figs, apricot should be soaked in water for 8 to 10 hours before they are taken orally.

17. Get Good Sleep

Sleep with health is happiness, nourishment, and strength. Sleep is important as eating healthy and exercising. Recent studies showed poor sleep is one of the risk factors for obesity, as it's linked to an 89% increased risk of obesity in children and 55% in adults. Quality sleep is essential for children's growth and development as it affects everything from body growth to mental functions. Studies have shown that children with an adequate amount of quality sleep have a better concentration, memory and overall mental and physical health.

18. Beat Food Addiction

A recent study found that 19.9% of people in North America and Europe fulfill the criteria for food addiction so beat this addiction of food.

19. Eat More Protein

Protein is an important nutrient for losing weight. Eating a high-protein diet to boost metabolism by 80–100 calories per day.

CHAPTER 14

Massage

"Massage is the only form of physical pleasure to which nature forgot to attach"

Body massage improves our health and removes much illness. Massage is a kind of exercise of muscles and by massage, blood flows in the small and thin blood vessels in the muscles. By massage, heat is generated in the blood which removes impurities in it and flushed out through sweat or urine. Hence, blood is purified and gives new energy and life to the body.

Mahatma Gandhi always had himself massaged for good health.

Mustard oil should be used for massage. Sprain and headache are relieved by massage. If there is paralysis in any part of the body, massage is giving a new life to it.

After the massage, the patient should take bath or his body wiped with a wet cloth. Massage arrests the aging of a person.

Body massage of small children naturally gives exercise to hands, feet, and stomach and the muscles of the chest. In villages, the newborn babies are given massage 2–3 times every day unlike in towns 1 time daily. After that, they are bathed in hot/lukewarm water and wiped by a dry towel. If small children are given regular massage they grow quickly and healthy.

The massage of old people is a form of exercise for them.

Scalp massage is similar to massage as of the back or body. Here fingertips of both hands applied light to medium pressure on the scalp in small circles. Oils used are peppermint oil or coconut oil or almond oil. You can apply oil on hair just before going to bed keeping old cloth/pillow or you can put oil when you are going to the office, school, or any other place.

Why Oil Message for Legs Benefits of Feet Oil Massage

Improves Blood Circulation

Our day goes into sitting and we rarely move around, especially during these lockdown days. This irregularity of walking and long hours of sitting can lead to improper blood circulation to our feet. To keep your feet healthy, all you need to do is take out 5 minutes for a oil massage. Just before sleeping massage your feet gently with any oil. If you are worried about the sheet getting stained, you can spread an old bedsheet below your feet.

Promotes Sleep

A good oil massage before bed helps in unwinding and relaxing as it gets rid of tension and relaxes your nerves. Your feet contain several acupuncture points that induce sleep. When you massage the whole of your foot, you also activate these acupuncture points. Hence, with increased blood circulation and relaxed nerves, a good night's sleep is ensured.

Eases Pain

Oil massage also soothes any kind of strain or pain in the feet. Massage the whole feet which helps in relaxing the muscles in your foot and relaxes your whole body for better sleep. It has been proved that massaging your feet with warm olive oil or coconut oil or sesame oil can provide relief from inflammation.

How to apply oil

1. Before sleeping, wash your feet with soap thoroughly.

2. Now sit on your bed with your legs spread in front.

3. Take a few drops of oil and massage your one feet at a time.

4. Massage with a firm hand and apply the oil on your soles, between the toes, and in the front.

5. Press each toe gently and stroke the length of your foot.

6. Continue doing the massage for more effectiveness.

7. Make sure you do this massage with slightly warm oil for deeper penetration.

8. Oils used are coconut, sesame, lavender, almond oil, and Olive Oil.

CHAPTER 15

No Smoking

"It is health that is the real wealth, and not pieces of gold and silver."

...Mahatma Gandhi

The Effects of Smoking on the Body

Smoking/tobacco is dangerous to your health. There are hazardous substances in any tobacco products example are nicotine and carbon monoxide. The substances you inhale will affect your lungs they can affect your entire body. Smoking can lead to a variety of complications in the body like

Central nervous system: One of the ingredients in tobacco is a intoxicating drug called nicotine which causes your brain in mere seconds and makes you feel more energized for a while. But as that effect wears off, you feel tired and crave for more cigarettes.

Respiratory system: When you inhale smoke, you're intaking substances that can damage your lungs like emphysema, the destruction of the air sacs in your lungs like chronic bronchitis , a group of lung diseases, lung cancer.

Cardiovascular system: Smoking damages your entire cardiovascular system as Nicotine causes blood vessels to tighten, and restricts the flow of blood. Smoking also raises blood pressure.

Digestive system: Smoking increases the risk of mouth, throat, larynx cancer.

CHAPTER 16

Joy of Giving

"Giving is the master key to success, in all applications of human life".

...Bryant McGill

Why Joy of Giving

Why joy of giving because it improves the health and overall wellbeing of the individual.

We get enjoyment through different means like listening to favorite music, watching films, spending time with family and friends, eating food, traveling, etc. In all these events, we are deriving enjoyment through those means which are centered on us and benefit us only.

There is the joy of giving, in which process though the giver loses something that belongs to him, yet he enjoys the moment because of the emotional fulfillment he derives when he helps his fellowmen who require help.

Mythological examples for the joy of giving: In our ancient mythology we find various examples of such selfless acts of giving like in Mahabharatha, Karna eldest brother of Pandavas was known or giving. He enjoyed this act of giving so much that he joyfully gave away the armor (Kavacha) and earrings (Kundala) that were attached to his body when Brahmin asked for them. He did not even bother to ask the Brahmin why he needed them and this cost his life.

Maya Angelou had said when we give then everyone is blessed when they give cheerfully and accept gratefully.

Other examples of Rich people: In the modern world to we find such great people who have given away large amounts of wealth purely for the joy of giving. Jeff Bezos (Amazon),Mark Zuckerberg (Facebook), Bill Gates(Microsoft), Warren Buffet, Ratan Tata (Tata Group), Azim Premji(Wipro), Mahindra company, Infosys, Shiv Nadar(HCL), Mukesh Ambani (Reliance Industries), Akshay Kumar (Filmstar), Virat Kohli (cricketer) have gained enormous riches. But they soon realized that amassing money did not give the same kind of enjoyment as that of giving it away to others and that is how they formed Foundations through which they have given away millions of dollars of money to the worthy causes.

To experience the joy of giving it is important that one has to have a tremendous amount of money even a small help to someone who is in need can bring joy to the giver and receiver. People who are happy by giving will experience real joy, health in their lives.

> *"If you knew what I know about the power of giving,*
> *You would not let a single meal pass without*
> *sharing it in some way."*

...Lord Buddha

Conclusion

"Thank you to all the people who have triggered my issues. You have helped me clarify what they are, start the healing process and ultimately become a better person."

...Renae A. Sauter

* * * * * * * *

And this brings us to the end of this book.

Now, you are equipped with all the understanding about how health works. You are well aware of many creative thinking techniques that can supply you with more than a handful of ideas to handle your health challenges in different areas of your life.

I wrote this book in a manner that you could use and implement health while reading the book. I hope you had taken out time alongside to do the required exercises and if yes, I'm sure you'd have already experienced a rise in your health abilities.

However, I understand that some people first want to understand the whole concept of health by reading the complete book before trying to implement that and you are in that category, no worries, you can now start revisiting the exercises and food to see the results for you.

Though I write my books specifically to add value to the lives of my readers (it's you!), but I always have some personal motive in my head to valuable insights while doing health research so that I can get benefitted by implementing them in my life.

Therefore, I invite you to this journey with me to practice what we just learned in the book and deepen our experience of life by experimenting with multiple health techniques.

To help you get a quick summary, I've captured all the big ideas of every health chapter with respective articles at the end of the book so that you can have a bird's eye view of the content.

If you want to remain Healthy

Give up	Adopt
Habit of eating without hunger	Fasting
Laziness	Hard work
Physical tiredness	Necessary rest
Mental tension, Selfishness	Prayer, Selflessness
Flour	Whole meal flour, sprouted wheat & pulses
Pickles	Salad
Fried vegetables	Raw or boiled vegetables
Soft drinks	Fruit, milk ,buttermilk and vegetable juice
Market sweets	Dry fruits like almond, raisins

As we all know, repetition is the mother of learning. So let's keep exposing our minds to the resourceful information on a regular basis, and let the compound effect work to our advantage in developing a creative mind and lead a healthier life of joy, abundance, and success. I wish you nothing but loads of success by generating and implementing great ideas in all your endeavors with regarding health and diet. I had increased my weight to 95 kilograms in the lockdown period that is march to may end 2020.So I took some important measures for my health. Then I took measures which are brought in following chapters. If you follow one chapter or all chapter you will definitely reduce weight as I have reduced from 95 kilograms to 85 kilograms (10 kilograms in 3 months) and my aim is to reduce still more kilograms as I was inspired by fitness of Indian captain Virat Kohli, Ranveer Singh, and, Dhoni.

Cheers May I ask you for a small favor?

At the outset, I want to give you a big thanks for taking out time to read this Lockdown health book. You could have chosen any other book, but you took mine, and I totally appreciate this.

I hope you got at least a few actionable insights that will have a positive impact on your day to day life.

Can I ask for 30 seconds more of your time?

I'd love if you could leave a **review** about the book. **Reviews** may not matter to big-name authors; but there are more valuable for authors like me, who don't have much following. They help me to grow my readership by encouraging folks to take a chance on my Health books.

To put it straight– **reviews are the life line for any author.**

Connect me on YouTube channel for road safety videos and incredible india videos

https://www.youtube.com/channel/UCaqqYeTd0lKMt1GYLglDg

Or search **Incredible india plus** in Google/youtube

Or watch Kailash temple with over 1,00,000 views

https://youtu.be/v7Be1k9E32g

Connect me on Instagram

drprashant_shetty or
drprashant10@rediffmail.com

Bibliography

1. A.Misra, U. Shrivastava Obesity and dyslipidemia in South Asians.

2. answersdrive.com

3. articles.bplans.com

4. Abs workouts. The Best Abs Workout: Circuits For Upper Abs, Lower Abs, And Obliques And Core. COACH

5. allure.vanguardngr.com

6. alivebynature.com

7. www.artofliving.org

8. artoflivingandscience.blogspot.com

9. www.authorstream.com

10. Astrand P, Rodahl K. Textbook of Work Physiology: Physiological Bases of Exercise. New York: McGraw-Hill, 1986.

11. Allen, Matthew. 'Rewriting the Script for South Asian Dance'. The Drama Review, 1997;41(3): 63–100.

12. Ashley Marcin. What are the top 12 benefits of swimming?2017 www.healthline.com.

13. Beth Bischoff CORE EXERCISES 30 Best Ab Workouts of All Time MENS JOURNAL.(Available on www.mensjournal.com health-fitness 30 – best-abs-exercise).

14. Brown RA, AbrantesAM, Minami H, et al. A preliminary, randomized trial of aerobic exercise for alcohol dependence. J Subst Abuse Treat. 2014;47(1):1–9.

15. Bateman LA, Slentz A, Willis LH, Shields AT, Piner LW, Bales CW, Houmard JA, and Kraus WE. Comparison of Aerobic Versus Resistance Exercise Training Effects on Metabolic Syndrome (from the Studies of a Targeted Risk Reduction Intervention Through Defined Exercise – STRRIDE-AT/RT). The American Journal of Cardiology. September 2011,837–844.

16. Booth FW, Roberts CK, Laye MJ. Lack of exercise is a major cause of chronic diseases. Compr Physiol. 2012;2(2):1143–1211.

17. Bayaz R. Aerobic exercise boosts brainpower. New York | Heidelberg, 13 December 2012.

18. www.business-standard.com

19. Boschmann M, Steiniger J, Franke G, Birkenfeld AL, Luft FC, Jordan J. Water drinking induces thermogenesis through osmosensitive mechanisms. J Clin Endocrinol Metab. 2007;92(8):3334–3337.

20. Baranowski, T., et al.: Assessment, prevalence, and cardiovascular benefits of physical activity and fitness in youth. Med Sci Sports Exerc 24: (supp) 5237–5247 (1992).

21. Brehm BJ, Seeley RJ, Daniels SR, D'Alessio DA. A randomized trial comparing a very low carbohydrate diet and a calorie-restricted low-fat diet on body weight and cardiovascular risk factors in healthy women. J Clin Endocrinol Metab. 2003;88(4):1617 – 1623.

22. www.betterhealth.vic.gov.au

23. Bhagvad gita book

24. blog.kismetnutrients.com

25. basicyogasana.blogspot.com

26. www.befantastico.com

27. www.capcana.com

28. www.coursehero.com

29. www.cmcmohali.com

30. www.curioushalt.com

31. colossal-sport-nutrition.com

32. Chen CK. Brisk Walking: The Underused Modality to Alleviate Obesity. J Obes Weight Loss Ther 2014;4: e112.

33. Clark LV, Pesola F, Thomas JM, Williamson MV, Beynon M, White PD. Guided graded exercise self-help plus specialist medical care versus specialist medical care alone for chronic fatigue syndrome (GETSET): a pragmatic randomized controlled trial. Lancet 2017; 390: 363–73.

34. Chaput JP, Klingenberg L, Rosenkilde M, Gilbert JA, Tremblay A, Sjödin A. Physical activity plays an important role in body weight regulation. J Obes. 2011;2011:360257

35. Chomentowski P, Dubé JJ, Amati F, et al. Moderate exercise attenuates the loss of skeletal muscle mass that occurs with intentional caloric restriction-induced weight loss in older, overweight to obese adults. J Gerontol A Biol Sci Med Sci. 2009;64(5):575–580.

36. Chen CK. Brisk Walking: The Underused Modality to Alleviate Obesity. J Obes Weight Loss Ther 2014;4: e112.

37. Connolly LJ, Nordsborg NB, Nyberg M, Weihe P, Krustrup P, Mohr M. Low-volume high-intensity swim training is superior to high-volume low-intensity training in relation to insulin sensitivity and glucose control in inactive middle-aged women. Eur J Appl Physiol. 2016;116(10):1889–1897.

38. Cappuccio FP; Taggart FM; Kandala NB; Currie A; Peile E; Stranges S; Miller MA. A meta-analysis of short sleep duration and obesity in children and adults. SLEEP 2008;31(5):619–626.

39. Charles Platkin.16 Tips So You Can Be Your Own Personal Trainer! DIET DETECTIVE.

40. https://www.coachmag.co.uk/workouts/abs-workouts

41. https://www.coachmag.co.uk/abs-workouts/5480/abs-workouts-for-the-gym-circuits-for-upper-abs-lower-abs-and-obliques-and-core

42. dailyhealthalerts.com

43. Dehghan M, Akhtar-Danesh N, Merchant AT.Childhood obesity, prevalence, and prevention.Nutr J. 2005;4:24. Published 2005 Sep 2.

44. www.dreamstime.com

45. Dennis EA, Dengo AL, Comber DL, et al. Water consumption increases weight loss during a hypocaloric diet intervention in middle-aged and older adults. Obesity (Silver Spring). 2010;18(2):300–307.

46. Dulloo AG, Geissler CA, Horton T, Collins A, Miller DS. Normal caffeine consumption: influence on thermogenesis and daily energy expenditure in lean and post obese human volunteers. Am J Clin Nutr. 1989;49(1):44–50.

47. Dulloo AG, Seydoux J, Girardier L, Chantre P, Vandermander J. Green tea and thermogenesis: interactions between catechin-polyphenols, caffeine, and sympathetic activity. Int J Obes Relat Metab Disord. 2000;24(2):252–258.

48. www.desilinks.co

49. www.desiakhbar.com

50. www.theeducationmagazine.com

51. www.eduofyoga.com

52. eddysatriya.wordpress.com

53. ebookbees.com

54. Ekeland E, Heian F, Hagen KB, Abbott J, Nordheim L. Exercise to improve self-esteem in children and young people. Cochrane Database Syst Rev. 2004;(1):CD003683.

55. Ekeland E, Heian F, Hagen KB. Can exercise improve self-esteem in children and young people? A systematic review of randomized controlled trials. Br J Sports Med. 2005;39(11): 792–798.

56. Elmagd MA. Benefits, need and importance of daily exercise. International Journal of Physical Education, Sports and Health 2016; 3(5): 22–27

57. www.finessyoga.com177.https://www.finessyoga.com/yoga-asanas/bhujangasana-step-precautions-benefits

58. www.fitsri.com

59. https://food.ndtv.com/beauty/10-foods-for-glowing-skin-1246425.

60. Friedenreich CM, Orenstein MR. Physical Activity and Cancer Prevention: Etiologic Evidence and Biological Mechanisms, The Journal of Nutrition, November 2002, Volume 132, Issue 11, Pages 3456S–3464S.

61. Foster, Susan Leigh (1997) 'Dancing Bodies'. In J. C. Desmond (ed.), Meaning in Motion: New Cultural Studies of Dance (pp. 235–58). Durham and London: Duke University Press.

62. GymGuider.com

63. www.ghpclinic.com

64. Griffin ÉW, Mullally S, Foley C, Warmington SA, O'Mara SM, Kelly AM. Aerobic exercise improves hippocampal function and increases BDNF in the serum of young adult males. Physiol Behav. 2011;104(5):934–941.

65. Guiney H, Machado L. Benefits of regular aerobic exercise for executive functioning in healthy populations. Psychon Bull Rev. 2013;20(1):73–86.

66. Gries KJ, Raue U, Perkins RK, Lavin KM, Overstreet BS, D'Acquisto LJ, Graham B, Finch WH, Kaminsky LA, Trappe TA, and Trappe S. Cardiovascular and skeletal muscle health with lifelong exercise. Journal of Applied Physiology.November 2018 Volume 125 Issue 5: Pages 1636–1645.

67. Gill JM, Sattar N. Fruit juice: just another sugary drink?.Lancet Diabetes Endocrinol. 2014;2(6):444–446.

68. Gupta S. Consume tulsi on an empty stomach for these 9 powerful benefits. (Google)

69. www.genengnews.com

70. Gita Ramesh. author The Ayurvedic Cookbook

71. getdownsized.com

72. www.gyanamrit.bkinfo

73. getfitkit.org

74. www.gov.uk

75. www.healthshots.com

76. Hyde, Colin, Vadnerkar, Smita, and Cutting, Angela (1996) Parampara—Continuing the Tradition: Thirty Years of Indian Dance and Music in Leicester. Leicester: Leicester City Council Living History Unit.

77. https://www.healthline.com/nutrition/weight-loss-herbs

78. https://www.healthifyme.com/blog/5-pranayamas-make-part-daily-fitness-schedule/

79. Höglund P, Nilsson LA.On running late in life. Arch Intern Med. 2009;169(7):719–720.

80. Hodgson AB, Randell RK, and JeukendrupAE.The Effect of Green Tea Extract on Fat Oxidation at Rest and during Exercise: Evidence of Efficacy and Proposed Mechanisms. Adv. Nutr.2013; 4: 129–140.

81. Hursel R, Viechtbauer W, Westerterp-Plantenga MS. The effects of green tea on weight loss and weight maintenance: a meta-analysis. Int J Obes (Lond). 2009;33(9):956–961.

82. Harris L, Hamilton S, Azevedo LB, et al. Intermittent fasting interventions for treatment of overweight and obesity in adults: a systematic review and meta-analysis. JBI Database System Rev Implement Rep. 2018;16(2):507–547.

83. Hunter GR, Byrne NM, Sirikul B, et al. Resistance training conserves fat-free mass and resting energy expenditure following weight loss. Obesity (Silver Spring). 2008;16(5):1045–1051.

84. Hunter GR, Byrne NM, Sirikul B, et al. Resistance training conserves fat-free mass and resting energy expenditure following weight loss. Obesity (Silver Spring). 2008;16(5):1045–1051.

85. https://www.healthshots.com/healthy-eating/superfoods/consume-tulsi-on-an-empty – stomach-for-these-9-powerful-benefits/

86. https://www.herzindagi.com/health/drink-masala-tea-health

87. www.herzindagi.com

88. www.happify.com

89. www.hbnindia.com

90. https://www.healthline.com/health/smoking/effects-on-body

91. https://www.hindujagruti.org/Hinduism-for   –kids/238_surya_namaskar.html

92. https://hohealthfitness.blogspot.com/2020/09/26-weight-loss-tips-that-are-actually.html

93. https://healthline.com/nutrition/26-evidence-based-weight-loss-tips

94. https://www.healthshots.com/healthy-eating/superfoods/consume-tulsi-on-an-empty-stomach-for-these-9-powerful-benefits

95. https://www.healthline.com/health/insomnia

96. www.harithayogshala.com

97. healthtopical.com

98. Hong HR, Jeong JO, Kong JY, et al. Effect of walking exercise on abdominal fat, insulin resistance, and serum cytokines in obese women. J Exerc Nutrition Biochem. 2014;18(3):277–285.

99. https://indianexpress.com/article/lifestyle/health/why-kadi-patta-juice-can-become-an   –   effective-weight-loss-remedy-6485128/

100. Ismail MN, Chee SS, Nawawi H, Yusoff K, Lim TO, James WP. Obesity in Malaysia. Obes Rev. 2002;3(3):203–208.

101. Ismail I, Keating SE, Baker MK, Johnson NA. A systematic review and meta-analysis of the effect of aerobic vs. resistance exercise training on visceral fat. Obes Rev. 2012;13(1):68–91.

102. www.independent.co.uk.com

103. www.indianepress.com

104. www.i-scholar.in

105. indiaculturetree.com

106. www.ijem.in

107. www.isha.sadhguru.com

108. journals.sagepub.com

109. jeanlaguerre.com

110. Jarrett-Macauley, Delia (1997) Review on South Asian Dance in England. London: Arts Council.

111. Kokkinos PF, Holland JC, Narayan P, Colleran JA, Dotson CO, Papademetriou V. Miles run per week, and high-density lipoprotein cholesterol levels in healthy, middle-aged men. A dose-response relationship. Arch Intern Med. 1995;155(4):415–420.

112. ketogenicreviews.com

113. www.keepinspiring.me

114. kemmannu.com

115. KnabAM, Shanely RA, Corbin KD, Jin F, Sha W, Nieman DC. A 45-minute vigorous exercise bout increases metabolic rate for 14 hours. Med Sci Sports Exerc. 2011;43(9):1643–1648.

116. Kmietowicz Zosia. Aerobic and resistance exercise can boost brain power in over 50s, review finds BMJ 2017; 357:j1969.

117. Kuo CH, Harris MB. Abdominal fat-reducing outcome of exercise training: Fat burning versus hydrocarbon source redistribution? Canadian Journal of Physiology and Pharmacology.March 2016; 94(7).

118. Lowe MR, Doshi SD, Katterman SN, and Feig EH. Dieting and restrained eating as prospective predictors of weight gain. Frontiers in psychology. September 2013; Volume 4: Article 577: 1–7

119. Li L, Men WW, Chang YK, Fan MX, Ji L, Wei GX. Acute aerobic exercise increases cortical activity during working memory: a functional MRI study in female college students. PLoS One. 2014;9(6):e99222..

120. Lee DC, Lavie CJ, Vedanthan R. Optimal dose of running for longevity: is more better or worse?. J Am Coll Cardiol. 2015;65(5):420–422.

121. Ludwig DS, Majzoub JA, Al-Zahrani A, Dallal GE, Blanco I, Roberts SB. High glycemic index foods, overeating, and obesity.Pediatrics. 1999;103(3): E26.

122. Leidy HJ, Tang M, Armstrong CL, Martin CB, Campbell WW. The effects of consuming frequent, higher protein meals on appetite, and satiety during weight loss in overweight/obese men. Obesity (Silver Spring). 2011;19(4):818–824.

123. Ludwig DS, Peterson KE, Gortmaker SL. Relation between consumption of sugar-sweetened drinks and childhood obesity: a prospective, observational analysis. Lancet. 2001;357(9255):505–508.

124. https://lifeseasons.com/how-to-lose-weight-and-maintain-weight-loss

125. Muecke L, Simons Morton B Huang IW, Parcel G. Is Childhood Obesity Associated with High Fat Foods and Low Physical Activity? Journal of school health. January 1992 Volume 62, Issue1:Pages 19–23.

126. Malia Frey MOTIVATION How to Be Your Own Personal Trainer. Veywell fit (website) June 22, 2019.

127. www.mensfitness.com

128. www.menjournals.com

129. mokemagnetic.com

130. https://www.mensjournal.com/health-fitness/7-best-barbell-exercises-strong – core/attack-your-core/

131. Mitchell R. Is physical activity in natural environments better for mental health than physical activity in other environments? Social Science & Medicine. August 2013; Volume 91:Pages 130–134.

132. meerabaiyoga.com

133. medicalyukti.blogspot.com

134. Moore SC, Patel AV, Matthews CE, Berrington de Gonzalez A, Park Y, et al. Leisure Time Physical Activity of Moderat to Vigorous Intensity and Mortality: A Large Pooled Cohort Analysis. PLoS Med.2012;9(11): e1001335.

135. Morris JN, Hardman AE. Walking to health [published correction appears in Sports Med 1997 Aug;24(2):96];23(5):306–332.

136. https://www.medicalnewstoday.com/articles/245588

137. www.musely.com

138. Surya namaskar,www.wikepedia.org

139. Neville C, Henwood T, Beattie E, Fielding E. Exploring the effect of aquatic exercise on behavior and psychological well-being in people with moderate to severe dementia: a pilot study of the Watermemories Swimming Club. Australas J Ageing. 2014;33(2):124 – 127.

140. nutritionj.biomedcentral.com

141. www.ndtv.com

142. m.food.ndtv.com

143. https://www.nhs.uk/news/lifestyle-and-exercise/physical-activity-reduces-stress/

144. www.omicsonline.org

145. onlineinfoindubaidirectory.blogspot.com

146. www.pininterest.com

147. Puetz TW, Flowers SS, O'Connor PJ. A randomized controlled trial of the effect of aerobic exercise training on feelings of energy and fatigue in sedentary young adults with persistent fatigue. Psychother Psychosom. 2008;77(3):167–174..

148. Przemysław Bąbel. Memory of pain induced by physical exercise, Memory.2016; 24:4, 548–559,

149. Parcel, G. S., et al.: School promotion of healthful diet and physical activity: impact on learning outcomes and self-reported behavior. Health Educ 1989 Q 16: 181–199

150. Parcel, G. S., et al.: School promotion of healthful diet and exercise behavior: an integration of organization change and school learning theory interventions. J School Health 57:150–156 (1987).

151. Pursey KM, Stanwell P, Gearhardt AN, Collins CE, Burrows TL. The prevalence of food addiction as assessed by the Yale Food Addiction Scale: a systematic review. Nutrients. 2014;6(10):4552–4590.

152. Purnima Singh Weight Loss Diet: Melting gourd soup like butter, belly-thigh, and waist fat, try this. Navbharat Times.

153. www.panlajakasthuri.in

154. www.pfizer.com

155. pubmed.ncbi.nlm.nih.gov

156. pinterest. 13 Quotes on the joy and importance of Giving | Joy quotes

157. https://www.quotes.net/authors/Renae+A.+Sauter or

158. Quotes." Quotes.net. STANDS 4 LLC, 2020. Web. 16 Sep. 2020.

159. <https://www.quotes.net/authors/Renae+A.+Sauter+Quotes>.

160. www.quotes.net

161. https://www.quora.com/What-is-the-best-workout-for-abs

162. Roveda E, Sciolla C, Montaruli A, Calogiuri G, Angeli A, Carandente F. Effects of endurance and strength acute exercise on night sleep quality. International Sport Med Journal, Vol.12 No.3, 2011, pp. 113–124.

163. R Flores. Dance for health: improving fitness in African American and Hispanic adolescents. Public Health Rep. 1995 Mar-Apr; 110(2): 189–193.

164. www.revistascientificas.udg.mx

165. Rai Aishwarya (2003) 'Bollywood Dancing', BBC 2 Documentary [Aired 22 October 2003]. London: BBC.

166. https://www.researchgate.net/publication/33585573_The_ Evaluation_of_Obesity_in_Malaysia.

167. https://www.researchgate.net/publication/263888297_ Obesity_Weight_Loss_Therapy_Brisk_Walking_The_Underused_ Modality_to_Alleviate_Obesity

168. https://www.researchgate.net/publication//7622299_ Childhood_Obesity_Prevalence_and_Prevention

169. https://runrepeat.com/what-running-does-to-you-body

170. runrepeat.com

171. repository-tnmgrmu.ac.in

172. rubun.info

173. www.stylecraze.com

174. www.scribd.com

175. search.barnesandnoble.com

176. www.science.gov

177. shirleytwofeathers.com

178. steppinupdanceco.ca

179. smartchoicedrugstore.com

180. S. Behla, A. Misra.Management of obesity in adult Asian Indians. Indian Heart Journal; July–August 2017, Volume 69, Issue 4, Pages 539–544.

181. Serdula MK, Ivery D, Coates RJ, et al. Do obese children become obese adults? A review of the literature.Preventive Medicine. 1993 Mar;22(2):167–177.

182. Science of Natural Life by Dr.Rakesh Jindal. (Arogya Sewa Prakashan Publisher, Modinagar, U.P).

183. www.sarvyoga.com

184. www.sweetsuerenity.com

185. Surya Namaskara.Divine Life Society (sivanandaonline.org) in 2011.

186. https://www.srisriravishankar.org

187. Shamlee Pathare.5 pranayamas that you should make a part of your daily fitness schedule September 14, 2020, in Yoga

188. https://www.stylecraze.com/articles/sudarshan-kriya-steps-and-benefits/

189. www.sarvyoga.com

190. www.self.com

191. SHAPE MAGAZINE

192. Stefan Brené, Astrid Bjørnebekk, ElinÅberg, Aleksander A Mathé, Lars Olson, Martin Werme. Running is rewarding and antidepressive, Physiology & Behavior. 2007, Volume 92, Issues 1–2: Pages 136–140.

193. Smits JAJ, Tart CD, Rosenfield D, and ZvolenskyMJ.The interplay between physical activity and anxiety sensitivity in fearful responding to CO2 challenge. Psychosom Med. 2011 July; 73(6): 498–503.

194. Steinberg H, Sykes EA, Moss T, Lowery S, LeBoutillier N, Dewey A. Exercise enhances creativity independently of mood. Br J Sports Med. 1997;31(3):240–245.

195. Sofis MJ, Carrillo A, Jarmolowicz DP. Maintained Physical Activity Induced Changes in Delay Discounting. Behav Modif.2017 Jul;41(4):499–528.

196. Schnohr P, O'Keefe JH, Marott JL, Lange P, Jensen GB. Dose of jogging and long-term mortality: the Copenhagen City Heart Study. J Am Coll Cardiol. 2015;65(5):411–419.

197. Szabo, A., &Ábrahám, J. (2013). The psychological benefits of recreational running: A field study. Psychology, Health & Medicine, 18(3), 251–261.

198. Sadi Khan. sadi@runrepeat.com.

199. Schroeder K, Ratcliffe SJ, Perez A, Earley D, Bowman C, Lipman TH. Dance for Health: An Intergenerational Program to Increase Access to Physical Activity. J PediatrNurs. 2017; 37:29–34.

200. Sheppard A, Broughton MC. Promoting wellbeing and health through active participation in music and dance: a systematic review. Int J Qual Stud Health Well-being. 2020;15(1):1732526.

201. Schulze MB, Manson JE, Ludwig DS, et al. Sugar-sweetened beverages, weight gain, and incidence of type 2 diabetes in young and middle-aged women.JAMA. 2004;292(8):927–934.

202. www.samuelthomasdavies.com

203. SakshitaKhosla. Lemon-Ginger Recipes for Weight Loss: 5 ingenious ways to use lemon and ginger to lose weight faster! or https://www.india.com/lifestyle/lemon-ginger-

204. https://www.india.com/lifestyle/lemon-ginger-recipes-for-weight-loss-5-ingenious-ways-to-use-lemon-and-ginger-to-lose-weight-faster-1764484/

205. www.sciam.co.in

206. www.shuttercock.com

207. SomBathla. Think out of the box book. www.sombathla.com

208. Tucker A. Start-Up Manual Key Fitness Terms Everyone Should Know Before They Step Foot In A Gym

209. A Textbook of Svasthavrtta by Dr. Mangalagowri.V.Rao (Chaukhambha publishers, Varanasi,(U.P)

210. .self magazine.

211. www.sucesssimplified.in

212. Textbook of Swasthavrtta by Dr. ManglagowriV.Rao. (ChaukhambhaOrientalia Publisher, Varanasi, U.P)

213. Thom G, Lean M. Is There an Optimal Diet for Weight Management and Metabolic Health?.Gastroenterology. 2017;152(7):1739–1751.

214. www.tribecacare.com

215. www.telegraphindia.com

216. teachersplus.yogajournal.com

217. theweightloss.blog

218. .https://tamilbrahmins.wordpress.com/2013/02/18/benefits-of-surya-namaskar

219. https://theindiangent.in/best-abs-workout-perfect-for-men

220. https://timeislyf.com

221. https://trainrunningacademy.com/235

222. http://www.tigerchung.com/running/index.html

223. https://topfithub.com/why-are-you-running

224. Unnikrishnan AG, Kalra S, Garg MK. Preventing obesity in India: Weighing the options. Indian J EndocrinolMetab. 2012;16(1):4–6.

225. Vedic – stories.blogspot.com

226. www.verywellfit.com

227. Victor N. Davich. 8-minute Meditation Expanded: Quiet Your Mind. Change Your Life. Kindle edition

228. Victoria H Stiles, Brad S Metcalf, Karen M Knapp, Alex V Rowlands. A small amount of precisely measured high-intensity habitual physical activity predicts bone health in pre – and postmenopausal women in UK Biobank, International Journal of Epidemiology, December 2017,

229. Vander Wal JS, Gupta A, Khosla P, Dhurandhar NV. Egg breakfast enhances weight loss. Int J Obes (Lond). 2008;32(10):1545–1551.

230. Veldhorst MA, Westerterp KR, van Vught AJ, Westerterp-Plantenga MS. Presence or absence of carbohydrates and the proportion of fat in a high-protein diet affect appetite suppression but not energy expenditure in normal-weight human subjects fed in energy balance. Br J Nutr. 2010;104(9):1395–1405.

231. https://viral-revival.com/pound-dropping-advice-everyone-should-try

232. Warburton DER, Nicol W, Bredin SSD. Health benefits of physical activity: the evidence. CMAJ 2006;174(6):801–9.

233. weighteasyloss.com

234. W. P. T. James. Handbook of Obesity: Etiology and Pathophysiology.

235. Wollseiffen, P., Schneider, S., Martin, L.A. et al. The effect of 6 h of running on brain activity, mood, and cognitive performance. Exp Brain Res.2016;234:1829–1836.

236. Wen H, Wang L. Reducing effect of aerobic exercise on blood pressure of essential hypertensive patients: A meta-analysis. Medicine (Baltimore). 2017;96(11):e6150.

237. WILLIAMS P T. Walking and Running are Associated with Similar Reductions in Cataract Risk. Medicine and Science in Sports and Exercise. Medicine & Science in Sports & Exercise: June 2013 – Volume 45 – Issue 6 – p 1089–1096

238. Waite LJ. The Demographic Faces of the Elderly.Popul Dev Rev. 2004;30(Supplement):3–16.

239. Weinheimer EM, Sands LP, Campbell WW. A systematic review of the separate and combined effects of energy restriction and exercise on fat-free mass in middle-aged and older adults: implications for sarcopenic obesity. Nutr Rev. 2010;68(7): 375–388.

240. World Health Organization (2014) Obesity: Situation and trends.

241. writemyessay.onlineessaywritinghelp.org

242. weightlossathometipps.blogspot.com

243. workoutbyrahul.blogspot.com

244. Wansink B, van Ittersum K. Portion size me: plate-size induced consumption norms and win-win solutions for reducing food intake and waste. J Exp Psychol Appl. 2013;19(4):320–332.

245. www.wikizero.com

246. en.wikipedia.org

247. http://weightlosstipsafter50.blogspot.com/2018/09/full-proved-weight-loss-tips.html

248. Yuan WX, Liu HB, Gao FS, Wang YX, and Kai-Rong Qin KR. Effects of 8-week swimming training on carotid arterial stiffness and hemodynamics in young overweight adults. Biomed Eng Online. 2016; 15(Suppl 2): 151.

249. Yoga the science magazine

250. www.yogateacherstrainingrishikesh.com

251. YOGA QUEST magazine

252. www.yogicwayoflife.com

253. www.101yogastudio.com

254. Zhang, Z., Chen, W. A Systematic Review of the Relationship Between Physical Activity and Happiness. J Happiness Stud 20, 1305–1322 (2019).

255. 10 minutes brisk walking each day in mid-life for health benefits and towards achieving physical activity recommendations. Published August 2017 PHE publications.